Systemic Homeostasis
and Poikilostasis in Sleep

Is REM Sleep a Physiological Paradox?

Systemic Homeostasis and **Poikilostasis** in **Sleep**

Is REM Sleep a Physiological Paradox?

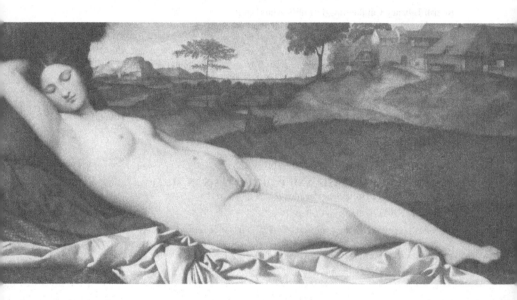

Pier Luigi Parmeggiani
University of Bologna, Italy

Imperial College Press

Published by

Imperial College Press
57 Shelton Street
Covent Garden
London WC2H 9HE

Distributed by

World Scientific Publishing Co. Pte. Ltd.
5 Toh Tuck Link, Singapore 596224
USA office: 27 Warren Street, Suite 401-402, Hackensack, NJ 07601
UK office: 57 Shelton Street, Covent Garden, London WC2H 9HE

British Library Cataloguing-in-Publication Data
A catalogue record for this book is available from the British Library.

Front cover: *The Sleeping Venus* (1510) by Giorgione/Tiziano. Gemäldegalerie Alte Meister. Dresden, Germany. (Reproduced with permission from Allgemeine Verwaltung, Foto/Reproduktion. Staatliche Kunstsammlungen, Dresden, Germany.)

Back cover: *The Nightmare* (1781) by Johann Heinrich Füssli. The Detroit Institute of Arts, Detroit, U.S.A. (Reproduced with permission from Bridgeman Art Library Ltd., W2 4PH London, U.K.)

ISBN-13 978-1-84816-572-4
ISBN-10 1-84816-572-2

Typeset by Stallion Press
Email: enquiries@stallionpress.com

Printed in Singapore.

This book is dedicated to my wife Luisa and our children Antonia, Alberto, Francesca, Andrea and Giovanni.

Contents

Acknowledgements

I am particularly indebted to the late Walter Rudolf Hess, the Swiss Nobel Laureate in Physiology, for influencing deeply my way of considering the integrative aspects of the somatic and autonomic control exerted by the central nervous system. It was on his suggestion that I started to study sleep physiology during my stay at the Department of Physiology of the University of Zurich, Switzerland. From then on sleep became a topic that constantly interested me in my scientific career.

I express my gratitude to my friends and collaborators during many years of research on sleep in the Department of Physiology of the University of Bologna, Italy. Their names are mentioned in the list of references. Pierluigi Lenzi deserves additional thanks for his creative technical advice.

I wish to acknowledge the scientifically fruitful and friendly relationship with Giorgio Affanni (University of Morón, Argentina), Véronique Bach (University of Picardy, France), Ralph Berger (U.C. Santa Cruz, U.S.A.), Michael Chase (U.C.L.A., U.S.A.), Craig Heller (Stanford University, U.S.A.), Werner Koella (University of Bern, Switzerland), Jean-Pierre Libert (University of Picardy, France), Birendra Mallick (Jawaharlal Nehru University, India), Dennis McGinty (V.A.G.L.A.H.S. and U.C.L.A., U.S.A.), Adrian Morrison (University of Pennsylvania, U.S.A.), John Orem (Texas Tech University, U.S.A.), Marisa Pedemonte (C.L.A.E.H. University, Uruguay), Hartmut Schulz (University of Erfurt, Germany), Ricardo Velluti (Republic University, Uruguay) and Ennio Vivaldi (University of Chile, Chile).

I am very grateful to my old friend Adrian Morrison for his generous assistance in the editing of this book. Much credit goes to him in this finished work; any errors of fact or interpretation are mine.

Preface

Rem tene, verba sequentur

(Cato, De Rhetorica, fr. 15, Jordan)

Sleep has fascinated and challenged the human mind across the centuries for obvious reasons. The cessation of environmental awareness and the insurgence of dreaming consciousness from the subjective viewpoint, and the motor and postural quiescence combined with depression of reactivity to external stimuli from the objective viewpoint, are characteristics of sleep that could not be overlooked. However, sleep became an issue of experimental research only in the nineteenth century, when the doctrine of *"Vitalism"* was definitively abandoned (see Bernard, 1865). This doctrine proposed that the functions of a living organism depend on a vital force neither mechanical nor chemical that is not explicable by the laws of physics and chemistry.

The work of Caton (1875) on the bioelectrical activity of rabbits' brains recorded by means of a galvanometer *"is all the more remarkable in that it was made about half a century before electronic amplification became available in the biological laboratory"* (Brazier, 1960, p. 195). Unfortunately, the recording of such activity by means of the galvanometer was impractical compared to modern electronic techniques. As a consequence, electroencephalography was used only in animal studies by a few researchers. This technique was not used in clinical studies of sleep until the work of Berger (1929) that demonstrated brain electrical potentials in humans many years later. This is an example of the historical implications of inadequate technical support of physiological research, which was clearly one of the causes for the retarded development of a precise relation of behavioural sleep to brain bioelectrical activity (see Rechtschaffen and Kales, 1968).

Interest in the mechanisms of sleep was also stimulated by the experiments of brain stem transections by Bremer (1935), which resulted in continuous synchronisation of the electroencephalogram that was characteristic of sleep as it was known at the time of his work. Bremer's reinforcement of the idea of sleep as a passive phenomenon as a result of a functional deafferentation of the brain was indirectly supported also by the fact that electrical stimulation of the brain stem by Moruzzi and Magoun (1949) elicited the electroencephalographic desynchronisation that is observed during wakefulness. This result brought forth the fundamental discovery of the reticular activating system underlying arousal and wakefulness.

The influence of the experimental set-up on the nature of physiological inferences is revealed by the contemporaneous contrasting tenets of passive and active sleep induction in the years prior to 1953. The theory considering sleep a passive phenomenon was based on the electroencephalographic evidence of the effects of brain stem transections and stimulation mentioned before. The theory considering sleep an active phenomenon, on the other hand, was based on behavioural, somatic and autonomic evidence produced by electrical stimulation of the diencephalon (Hess, 1944; Parmeggiani, 1962), the limbic system (Parmeggiani, 1960, 1962), and the basal forebrain (Sterman and Clemente, 1962). These experiments suggested that the behaviour of sleep in mammals depends on the activation of a complex set of neuronal structures, including the limbic system (pre-sleep behaviour), in addition to those underlying the typical electroencephalographic changes. In fact, the drawback of emphasising the study of the bioelectrical activity of the brain was for a while an unintentional reductionist attitude towards physiological regulation during sleep. Other aspects of sleep, which make up its whole, were essentially ignored.

The synchronised electroencephalogram was considered equivalent to sleep until the existence of a sleep state characterised by electroencephalographic desynchronisation could no longer be overlooked (Aserinsky and Kleitman, 1953). The electroencephalographic dichotomy of sleep was later substantiated by the study of the dichotomy in sleep of physiological functions, such as postural control, thermoregulation, circulation and respiration. Eventually, the distinction between two basically different modalities of systemic physiological regulation gained fundamental relevance also for the development of sleep medicine.

This book is aimed at presenting biologists and clinicians with a concise description of the physiological phenomenology of sleep from the viewpoint of the principle of homeostasis, an issue that has not been fully appreciated as yet by basic and medical sleep research. In the jargon of the physiological literature, the word "*homeostasis*", proposed by W. B. Cannon in 1926, essentially means that a constant state of the extra-cellular body fluids exists with regard to their physical and chemical properties. Since normal cell function depends on a specific composition of such fluids in multi-cellular animals, there are many systemic regulatory mechanisms under the control of the central nervous system that act to maintain the constancy of the cellular environment. The experimental study of homeostasis had early on revealed to physiologists the nature and complexity of the underlying physiological regulation. Many of its mechanisms trigger compensatory changes according to the principle of negative feedback. However, the neural control of homeostasis still deserves full clarification with regard to its functional significance in sleep.

From a schematic viewpoint, it is necessary to divide the behavioural continuum in terms of consciousness into four states at least. According to the most general physiological features of such states, they may be called active wakefulness, quiet wakefulness, quiet sleep and active sleep.

Active wakefulness is characterised by a desynchronised electroencephalogram, prevalence of sympathetic activity and by skeletal muscle activity during different behaviours, such as orienting, exploring, feeding, mating, defence or attack. In this state, the organism may even temporarily incur a homeostatic debt depending on significant quantitative changes in the controlled physiological variables (e.g., O_2, CO_2, H^+) when the regulation exerted by the homeostatic mechanisms is overwhelmed by the catabolic request of intense skeletal muscle activity. The state of active wakefulness is therefore unsuitable for a balanced functional comparison with the metabolic condition of sleep, which is lowest in quiet sleep.

Leaving out active wakefulness, then, the physiological phenomena conventionally selected in adult mammals to identify the other behavioural states are here briefly outlined. They are: (i) desynchronised electroencephalogram, presence of postural muscle tone and stable activity of autonomic functions with slight sympathetic prevalence in quiet wakefulness; (ii) synchronised electroencephalogram, decrease in postural muscle tone, slow eye movements and stable activity of autonomic functions with parasympathetic prevalence in quiet sleep; (iii) desynchronised electroencephalogram, postural muscle atonia, myoclonic twitches and jerks, rapid eye movements and variable autonomic sympathetic and parasympathetic activity in active sleep.

Concerning the two sleep states, quiet and active, the most common names NREM sleep (also called: non-rapid-eye-movement [NREM] or synchronised or slow-wave sleep) and REM sleep (also called: rapid-eye-movement [REM], desynchronised, fast wave or paradoxical sleep) are adopted in this book.

This book brings forth experimental evidence demonstrating that the two states of sleep differ radically with respect to the short-term systemic regulation of many physiological variables underlying cellular life: homeostatic regulation is operative in NREM sleep and suspended in REM sleep. On this basis, these two states of sleep in mammals deserve the designations of *"homeostatic"* and *"poikilostatic"*, respectively. These qualifications point out the state-related persistence (static) of the functional action of the two modalities (*homeo* = integrated physiological functions and *poikilo* = disintegrated physiological functions) of systemic physiological regulation. The book also proposes to discuss the theoretical and functional importance of the principle of homeostasis as the fundamental criterion for the systematic characterisation of sleep-state dependent changes of the integrative control of physiological functions exerted by the central nervous system during sleep in mammals.

Early in the course of my experimental studies and later during the writing of the book, I have crossed several disciplinary borders of physiology as a way of approaching knowledge of the relevant issues in the context of the somatic and autonomic behaviour of sleep. In doing so, it was necessary to select issues and experimental data to bring forth an overall but essential picture of the complex functional framework that underlies such behaviours. The selection was necessarily limited to the physiological events occurring within the temporal boundaries of NREM sleep and REM sleep states.

The book is in part based on several reviews I have written over the years dealing with many physiological aspects of sleep. Many of the experimental results presented derive directly from the work of my laboratory in the Department of Human and General Physiology of the University of Bologna (Italy). Moreover, I highlight early contributions of other sleep researchers that were instrumental in opening at that time a new field of physiology in sleep (for additional references see also Parmeggiani, 1980a,b). In this connection, I take the responsibility for involuntary omissions.

It is my hope that the book may also contribute to the preservation of the memory of a conceptually exciting and experimentally rewarding epoch of sleep research and to draw new generations of scientists to the study of sleep physiology and sleep medicine.

Chapter 1

The Principle of Homeostasis

In the jargon of physiology, the word "*homeostasis*", introduced by W. B. Cannon (1926) into the physiological literature, means that a state of constancy exists in the physical and chemical properties in extra-cellular body fluids. Historically, C. Bernard (1878) is credited with having pointed out the "*fixité*" of the "*milieu interiéur*" as a central issue of physiology. Both pioneers opened up and sustained a new field of research that is basic in systems physiology, particularly with regard to "*the integrative questions of order and control*" of physiological variables (Noble and Boyd, 1993, p. 12).

Cannon's interest (1929) in the issue promoted the experimental study of physiology according to this principle. He was aware of the necessity of supporting the theory with a deep knowledge of the underlying physiological mechanisms. His endeavour substantially clarified the significance of the principle of homeostasis from the functional viewpoint and revealed the great complexity of the mechanisms involved in "*the integrated co-operation of a wide range of organs*". He expressed the confidence that "*homeostasis is not accidental but is a result of organized government, and that search for the governing agencies will result in their discovery*" (Cannon, 1929, p. 426).

Cannon advanced propositions of general criteria according to which physiological mechanisms maintain steady states in the organism. It is worthwhile quoting two more of his concise statements (Cannon, 1929, pp. 424 and 425). "*In an open system such as our bodies represent, compounded of unstable material and subjected continually to disturbing conditions, constancy is in itself evidence that agencies are acting, or ready to act, to maintain this constancy.*"

Furthermore, "*If state remains steady it does so because any tendency towards change is automatically met by increased effectiveness of the factor or factors which resist the change*". Cannon's concept was, therefore, based on the physiological achievement of an enduring stability of the organism.

Functional Aspects of the Principle of Homeostasis

From a teleological viewpoint, the principle of homeostasis is key to appraising the role of physiological functions in the coupled context of the internal (organism) and the external environment. In other words, homeostasis reveals the success of physiological adjustments to endogenous and exogenous influences challenging the harmony of a balanced interaction between organism and environment in the temporal continuum of life. For reasons that will be detailed in the next chapter (see Chapter 2, section: Practical criteria for the study of systemic homeostasis and poikilostasis in sleep), a general limit is set to this study. The verification of the principle of homeostasis in this book concerns the physiology of systemic functions (systemic homeostasis). In addition, also the processes underlying the compartmentalised homeostasis in the brain of two physiological variables (temperature and blood flow) are taken into consideration in Chapter 7.

Almost axiomatic today is the concept that the maintenance of the constancy of physical and chemical variables in the extra-cellular compartment of the organism depends on physiological mechanisms operating under the integrative control of the central nervous system. The result of this control is that the disturbing effects of a variety of exogenous (environment) or endogenous (organism) influences are continuously monitored and counteracted to maintain a stable physiological condition of the extra-cellular fluid. Were such effects unchallenged, the constancy in composition of the extra-cellular fluid would be modified to the detriment of normal cellular life. For this reason, variables of the arterial blood and interstitial fluid with regard to temperature, hydrogen ion, oxygen and carbon dioxide, water, electrolytes, glucose, etc. are considered here as *fundamental* in the context of this general approach to the principle of homeostasis.

It is important to realise that belief in a quantitative constancy of the fundamental variables in the extra-cellular body fluids, though valid theoretically, is only approximately true. In normal physiological conditions, the fundamental variables that are compartmentalised in the different body tissues and organs continuously oscillate within small quantitative ranges. Such oscillations are not only compatible with, but also the true expression of the processes underlying normal cellular life. In addition, the slow oscillations with circadian rhythmicity are also physiologically normal and are controlled by the circadian clock located in the anterior hypothalamic area (suprachiasmatic nucleus).

Deviations of the fundamental variables beyond the physiological range elicit error signals in receptors (thermo-, baro-, chemo-, mechano- and nociceptive) influencing the central nervous system. As a result, somatic, autonomic and endocrine physiological responses are elicited in order to return the fundamental variables to their normal ranges.

In terms of control theory, the changes in both the fundamental variables of the organism and the ambient cues influence feedback (reactive homeostatic) and feedforward (predictive homeostatic) mechanisms, respectively, adjusting the control systems of other variables that are *instrumental* in the maintenance of the homeostasis of the fundamental variables. These two different kinds of regulation are controlled and modulated by the integrative action of the central nervous system, which activates somatic, autonomic and endocrine effector mechanisms, and also adjusts set point and gain of feedback and feed forward mechanisms when necessary. The efferent activity that influences fundamental variables, is tuned up during wakefulness, due to a large variety of endogenous and exogenous challenges, and periodic ambient cues. Tuning is different during sleep as a result of stereotyped changes lowering the responsiveness of the central nervous system to internal and external stimuli. Moreover, the protective postures of sleep and the choice of favourable sleep sites decrease the disturbing influence of ambient stimulation. Auditory processing is the least affected by sleep (see Velluti, 2008). It is also modulated in connection with parental duties or specific environmental dangers.

As indicated above, in addition to the "reactive mode" of homeostatic control, there is also a "predictive mode" (see Moore-Ede, 1986, for terminology and conceptual definition). Predictive homeostasis counteracts in advance future disturbing influences with the result being prevention or attenuation of energetically expensive and physiologically hampering responses of reactive homeostasis. For instance, circulatory and respiratory activity is enhanced just before the increase in the metabolic request for voluntary muscle work. In this case, predictive homeostasis copes at least partly with forthcoming disturbing influences of the metabolic demands of exercise on the constancy of fundamental variables. On an extended time scale, periodic ambient cues (e.g., light–dark or temperature seasonal changes) promote long-term qualitative and quantitative physiological provisions to prepare in advance the defence of the organism against the oncoming environmental challenges. By reducing their impact, predictive homeostasis improves the effectiveness of physiological responses and decreases the energy expenditure of reactive homeostasis. An example of predictive homeostasis, pertaining to the issues of this book, is the sleep posture assumed at sleep onset. Different postures favour selectively either body heat loss or conservation during NREM sleep depending on ambient temperature (see Chapter 5).

Two other forms of homeostatic control, namely *rheostasis* and *allostasis*, have been proposed. In rheostasis, the regulated levels are changed within definite intervals of time as a result of controlled oscillations in regulatory set points (e.g., slowly changing influences, such as circadian drives) (Mrosovsky, 1990). In allostasis, the predictive behavioural and physiological adjustments also induce physiological strain and eventually breakdown of regulation due to stress (Schulkin, 2003). Both mechanisms are not considered in this context since they do not fit into the short temporal frame of the ultradian sleep cycle (see Chapter 2).

Conceptual Dissection of Homeostasis: Physiological Parameters and Operators

Conceptually, the fundamental variables are the link between the efferent and afferent branches (neural or humoral) of feedback regulatory loops. The existence of such variables under constraining conditions of physiological optimisation suggests consideration of the fundamental variables as "parameters" that parametrise and quantify the functional state of the control systems of the whole organism. Thus, the term *"physiological parameters"* will be used in this book to refer to the fundamental variables. In turn, the instrumental variables (at systemic and molecular levels) are the executive operators of functions like circulation, respiration, thermoregulation, etc., which are continuously adjusted by the integrative control of the nervous system so as to maintain the approximate constancy of the physiological parameters. On this basis, the term *"physiological operators"* will be used in this book.

Physiological homeostasis depends on the action of systemic physiological operators that result from the combination of many subordinate physiological operators. In order to clarify this concept, two short elementary lists of subordinate physiological operators of two systemic operators, circulation and respiration, are outlined as follows. For example, the list concerning the measurable subordinate operators of circulation consists of the heart's contractility, stroke volume, rate and output, blood pressure, arterial conductance and flow, venous return, etc. Concerning respiration, the list consists of breathing rate, tidal volume, ventilation, diffusion of respiratory gases, pulmonary blood flow, etc. It is not redundant at this point to state again that the recruitment and control of the physiological operators of systemic functions is the result of the integrative action of the nervous system.

Dissecting the Physiological Phenomena of Sleep

Cannon was confident that *"homeostasis is not accidental but is a result of organized government, and that search for the governing agencies will result in their discovery"* (Cannon, 1929, p. 426). This search implies also the study of the neural mechanisms of the control of homeostasis during sleep.

In this book, the study regards the systemic homeostatic functions of respiration, circulation and thermoregulation. To this end, the spontaneous changes in the activity of the operators of such functions during sleep are evaluated with respect to homeostasis. In addition, also the experimental testing of the homeostatic significance of the responses of such operators to artificial stimulation during sleep will be considered.

Undoubtedly, there are also compartmentalised processes of direct and short-term regulation of physiological parameters in organs and tissues. For instance, the supply of oxygen from arterial blood to tissues depends not only on the partial pressure gradient maintained by the systemic respiratory and circulatory operators that support the delivery and removal of respiratory gases to and from cellular tissues. This exchange is also influenced at the haemoglobin level by several physiological parameters, such as carbon dioxide, hydrogen ion, and temperature, acting reciprocally also as operators in the capillaries. Also, the control of the hydrogen ion in blood is obtained by the interaction of many physiological parameters (e.g., oxygen, carbon dioxide, bicarbonate, chloride, haemoglobin and temperature) in connection with the systemic respiratory, circulatory and renal operators. At molecular levels, therefore, there is in many cases a *parameter-operator dualism* in function. The compartmentalisation of homeostatic mechanisms is considered in Chapter 7 concerning the brain as a special case.

Conclusion and Perspectives

The study of homeostasis in this book is limited to systemic functions that reveal clear differences in the neural control of their physiological operators during the sleep states. The lack of completeness of such data is not an obstacle to answering the question of whether the principle of systemic homeostasis applies to all behavioural states. This notion is a result of the appraisal of the level of congruence of a sufficient number of systemic physiological events that support the life of a normal organism.

The following chapters show that the physiological consistency of the principle of homeostasis has been established as far as the integrative control of physiological functions by the central nervous system during NREM sleep. In contrast, many physiological events of REM sleep are quite inconsistent with the logic of the neural control of homeostasis. This condition of non-homeostatic neural regulation (poikilostasis) is an unresolved and important physiological issue, particularly concerning the teleological significance of the function of sleep.

Historically, the study of thermoregulation during sleep demonstrated for the first time a dramatic change in homeostatic neural regulation in a sleep state, namely, the lack of thermoregulation during REM sleep (Parmeggiani and Rabini, 1967). This result provided a good reason to explore also the basic, short-term survival functions, namely respiration and circulation, that are also involved in thermoregulation (see Parmeggiani, 1980a). Less dramatic but nevertheless appreciable differences between sleep states exist in the regulation of these functions. This book, therefore, deals with respiration and circulation during sleep and aims to define the temporal boundaries within which the principle of homeostasis is consistent or inconsistent not only with thermoregulation, but also with the regulation of these basic functions across the temporal continuum of sleep states.

Chapter 2

The Study of Homeostasis in Sleep

Introducing now the essential phenomenal aspects of sleep is a necessary step to understand its relationship with physiological homeostasis. Sleep is a sequence of behavioural states in response to a neuro-humoral clock mechanism influenced by several endogenous (feeding, fatigue, temperature, instinctive drives) and exogenous (light/dark cycle, temperature, food, season, social drives) cues. From the behavioural viewpoint, sleep appears so complex and multiform in nature as to defy any simple definition and justify a theoretical distinction between proximate (physiological phenomena), intermediate (neural control) and remote (genetic control) aspects of its determination (Parmeggiani, 2005a). Considering these factors in approaching the genesis of sleep avoids the rigid causal determination that would force sleep into a non-realistic reductionist theory. In fact, the elementary physiological events characterising sleep behaviour are not always specific to sleep alone. Sleep, like wakefulness, may be considered a "super-function" as a result of subordinate interactive functions. In normal conditions, it is not induced by the compelling influence of a segregated and highly specific neuronal network of the central nervous system (i.e., sleep centre). In general, wake and sleep behaviours may be considered the result of shifts in the functional dominance of phylogenetically different structures of the encephalon under the control of permissive influences of circadian pacemakers activated by organic and ambient cues.

Ultradian Sleep Cycle

The "*ultradian sleep cycle*" schematically consists of the sequence of two basic behavioural states that are conventionally named non-rapid-eye-movement (NREM) sleep (also called: synchronised, slow-wave sleep) and rapid-eye-movement (REM) sleep (also called: desynchronised, paradoxi-cal sleep). The differences in the bioelectrical (synchronised or desynchronised) activity of the brain measured by the electroencephalo-gram (EEG) as well as the absence or presence of rapid eye movements define conventionally the states. NREM sleep is characterised by a syn-chronised (relatively high amplitude and low frequency waves) electroencephalogram and REM sleep by a desynchronised (relatively low amplitude and high frequency waves) electroencephalogram. Further sub-division (sleep with spindle and slow wave electroencephalogram in animals and I, II, III, IV NREM stages in humans; tonic and phasic REM sleep stages in all species) of the two basic states is not always necessary for the present study of homeostasis in sleep. In particular, tonic REM sleep events are persistent as the desynchronised electroencephalogram and skeletal muscle atonia, whereas phasic REM sleep events are intermittent as rapid eye movements and muscle twitches. Repetition of this ultradian sleep cycle comprises the sleep periods of the daily wake–sleep sequences as circadian sleep cycle, which varies according to species. From the viewpoint of this book, the ultradian cycle of sleep is at the core of the problem of the neural control of homeostasis.

Circadian Sleep Cycle

Only a schematic description of the circadian organisation of the ultradian sleep cycle is presented here. The single sequence of NREM sleep and REM sleep episodes is the elementary temporal organisation of sleep that is replicated to constitute the circadian cycle of sleep in adult mammals. There are many kinds of circadian electroencephalographic and behav-ioural sleep patterns in the different species and at different ages, though, that will not be considered in detail here.

In the circadian framework, the ultradian sleep cycle occurs with a periodicity displayed throughout the day (polyphasic-distributed) or limited to either the light or dark hours of the day (polyphasic-clustered). In humans and some primates, the clustering of the cycles may be so tight in adulthood that intermingled wakefulness may be almost unnoticeable because it is usually so short lasting. In this case, the sleep pattern is called monophasic, if it occurs only during a period of the day (e.g., during the night), or diphasic, if it occurs in two temporally separated periods (e.g., nocturnal sleep and diurnal napping).

A pertinent question in this context is whether such different circadian organisations of the basic behavioural pattern of the ultradian sleep cycle are related to the homeostatic neural regulation of physiological functions. In particular, the architecture of the ultradian sleep cycle and its different circadian clustering in mammalian species is a complex result of bodily and ambient cues. Also the phylogenetic developments of different mechanisms of homeostatic neural regulation of the physiological parameters and particularly of body core temperature play a role. The latter variable strongly and directly affects the physiological and biochemical processes because it is a specific (thermoregulation) and a non-specific (according to the Q_{10} law) regulator of the energy flow in the organism.

Suspension of the Systemic Control of Homeostasis in REM Sleep

The tenet that mammalian species are endowed with a steadily active neural control of homeostasis across wakefulness and sleep had not been systematically tested until the second part of the nineteenth century when REM sleep became a hot issue in neurophysiology. Before that time, it was common knowledge that homeostasis of several physiological parameters is not fully achieved during the state of active wakefulness, e.g., during muscular exercise. Accordingly, it was not conceivable that homeostasis could be challenged during the motor quiescence of sleep. Only the discovery of REM sleep (Aserinsky and Kleitman, 1953) and the subsequent study of its physiology, and particularly of thermoregulation (Parmeggiani and Rabini, 1967), produced the experimental evidence that this state of sleep is quite different in the neural control of physiological parameters compared with both wakefulness and NREM sleep (see Parmeggiani, 1980a).

Concerning wakefulness, for instance, it is well known that intense muscular effort with the prevalence of anaerobic glycolysis may temporarily bring about an increasing loss of homeostatic compensation (e.g., metabolic acidosis). Quite rightly, however, it was appreciated that in such conditions homeostatic mechanisms are still active and only temporarily and quantitatively overwhelmed by the metabolic effects of muscular exercise. At the onset of skeletal muscle activity, the early increases in respiratory and circulatory activity, due to proprioceptive reflexes and central neural mechanisms, tend to compensate for incoming metabolic loads. In addition, there is a regulated early increase in body temperature, which also underlies positive thermophysical and thermochemical influences (according to the Q_{10} law) improving the metabolic energy transformation into work. Later on during exercise, the excess of heat produced is disposed of by efficient thermoregulation. During intense muscle exercise, circulatory and respiratory compensation for the increasing homeostatic debt, due to the metabolic acidosis elicited by anaerobic glycolysis, is also important. In conclusion, it is justified to think that a variety of both short and long term mechanisms of homeostasis are at work in wakefulness, enacting Cannon's pregnant expression of *"the wisdom of the body"* (Cannon, 1932).

The issue of a "constitutional" impairment of homeostatic regulation during sleep was first raised by the study of thermoregulation in cats exposed to negative (cold) and positive (warm) ambient thermal loads with respect to the neutral ambient temperature of the species. The unexpected observation (Fig. 1) was that in the cat two important thermoregulatory

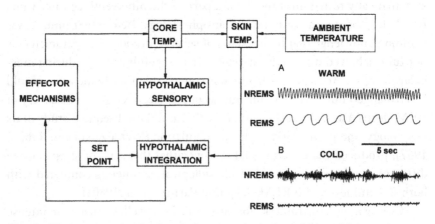

Fig. 1. Tachypnea and shivering during sleep (cat). A: at high ambient temperature (warm: 37°C), the pneumogram shows the presence of tachypnea during NREMS and the absence during REMS. B: at low ambient temperature (cold: 6°C) the electromyogram of the neck muscles shows that the bursts of shivering activity are present during NREMS and absent during REMS. NREMS, NREM sleep; REMS, REM sleep. (Modified from Parmeggiani and Rabini, 1967.)

responses, tachypnea and shivering, are present in NREM sleep and absent in REM sleep.

This unquestionable evidence of a dichotomy in the response to thermal loads depending on sleep states was the beginning of a series of studies of both peripheral and central mechanisms controlling thermal homeostasis during the ultradian sleep cycle. The existence of a clear-cut suppression of thermoregulation during REM sleep was clearly established particularly in furry mammalian species of small body size. In addition, other remarkable regulatory differences between the two sleep states were then observed with regard to postural, circulatory, respiratory and autonomic functions in general (see Parmeggiani, 1980a). The clear conclusion was that a basic dichotomy in systemic physiological regulation characterises NREM sleep and REM sleep in terms of two opposite modalities of neural control, i.e., *homeostatic* and *poikilostatic*, respectively. These qualifications point out the state-related persistence (static) of the functional action of the two modalities (*homeo* = integrated physiological functions and *poikilo* = disintegrated physiological functions) of the systemic physiological regulation.

This striking functional dichotomy of sleep in mammals means that the poikilostatic control of physiological operators during REM sleep is a normal physiological event since it does not alter so dangerously the physiological parameters so as to affect normal health conditions and, ultimately, the survival of the species. The main reason is that the duration of this state of sleep is in general shorter than the time required for a massive transfer of the effects of the poikilostatic control of physiological operators to the physiological parameters underlying the short-term survival conditions of body tissues. This assumption is particularly appealing concerning thermoregulation. In species with different body mass (e.g., rats, rabbits, cats, humans) the average duration of REM sleep episodes increases with the increase in body and brain weight, a determinant of the thermal inertia. Such inertia delays the changes in body core temperature so alarming as to elicit arousal from REM sleep. In addition, other factors, such as fur, food and predator–prey relationships influencing REM sleep duration ought also to be mentioned here. The arousal from REM sleep supports in general the maintenance of homeostasis, since this response is the quickest and best defence against dangerous drifts of physiological parameters by restoring the full somatic and autonomic control of homeostasis by the nervous system.

Practical Criteria for the Study of Systemic Homeostasis and Poikilostasis in Sleep

Two general criteria underlie the selection of the physiological phenomena considered in this book. The first is that *the time constants of the functions under scrutiny ought to fit the temporal dimensions of the states of the ultradian sleep cycle.* The second is that *the analysis of functions may be restricted to the systemic physiological operators.*

These criteria help us to take a short cut across the "forest" of experimental obstacles that would hamper the direct study of a large number of physiological parameters. An additional difficulty for the analysis is particularly evident when taking into account the problem, mentioned in the previous chapter, of the existence in many cases of a parameter–operator dualism in the functional role of the same variable.

Systemic Dissection and Recombination of Physiological Functions

In this context, the dissection of the physiological functions consists of the analysis of the specific physiological operators during sleep in both natural and artificial conditions. In natural conditions, it is possible to observe that the spontaneous respiratory, muscular and vasomotor responses of thermoregulation to ambient thermal load are present in NREM sleep and lacking in REM sleep. In artificial conditions, the stimulation (electrical, thermal) of neural structures underlying the control of such responses is used to verify the previous results. For instance, by means of direct thermal stimulation of preoptic-anterior hypothalamic thermoregulatory structures tachypnea was obtained only during NREM sleep (Fig. 2).

The conceptual recombination of all the data collected on the basis of the physiological dissection of functions is necessary to infer whether or not a systemic neural control of the physiological operators is actually operative according to either the homeostatic or the poikilostatic mode. For instance, in NREM sleep, a stable decrease in heart rate, cardiac

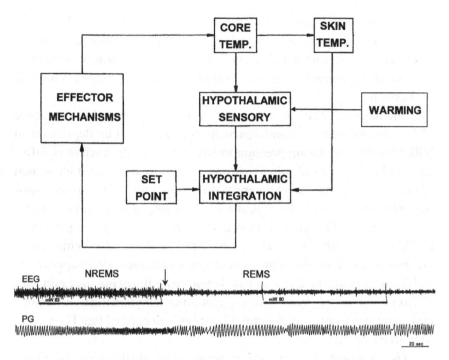

Fig. 2. Respiratory effects of preoptic-anterior hypothalamic diathermic warming during sleep (cat). Warming elicits tachypnea during NREMS and is ineffective during REMS. Note that the tachypnea disappears immediately at the beginning of REMS. EEG, electroencephalogram; mW, milliwatt; PG, pneumogram; NREMS, NREM sleep; REMS, REM sleep. (Modified from Parmeggiani *et al.*, 1973.)

stroke volume and output, arterial blood pressure, breathing frequency and a quiescent thermoregulatory lying posture associated with a slight decrease in core temperature is observed. All this is consistent with a homeostatically regulated functional equilibrium of the postural, circulatory, respiratory, thermoregulatory mechanisms in a condition of decreased metabolic rate. Inconsistent with a goal-directed autonomic activity are the following functional features of REM sleep: irregular heart rate, variable cardiac stroke volume and output, variable arterial pressure and irregular breathing rate. Concerning the somatic activity in REM sleep, the loss of protective posture, according to the thermal conditions, associated with irregular twitches and jerks of atonic muscles that are due to phasic random activation during tonic inhibition of motoneurons (see Chase and Morales, 2005), is also functionally incon-sistent. Such irregular and contradictory influences on motoneurons are rather consistent with a poikilostatic state. In conclusion, it is hard to extrapolate a coherent functional purpose from such phenomenology in REM sleep.

The neuronal circuits underlying sleep promotion and the sequence of behavioural states are only partially understood. The depression in NREM sleep and the suppression in REM sleep of the excitatory influence on brain stem and spinal neurons exerted by the regulatory system of the excitatory neuromodulator orexin/hypocretin located in the hypothalamus (Peyron *et al.*, 1998) probably play a role to promote and sustain sleep processes. This effect is associated with GABAergic and galaninergic inhibition (Sherin *et al.*, 1998), starting from the ventrolateral preoptic nucleus, of the neurons active in wakefulness (see Saper *et al.*, 2001). As a result, the activity of such neurons influencing the brain with different excitatory transmitters (serotonin, noradrenaline, histamine, glutamate, aspartate, acetylcholine) is strongly depressed (see Brown and McCarley, 2005).

The existence of a switch mechanism of the modality of the central integrative control of thermoregulation (Parmeggiani *et al.*, 1973), respiration (Parmeggiani, 1978, 1979) and circulation (Azzaroni and Parmeggiani, 1993) at onset and end of REM sleep was early documented by the quick phenomenal transitions of such functions.

The neuronal network underlying the operation of such a switch is at present under scrutiny. A group of researchers (Lu *et al.*, 2006) has suggested that GABAergic REM-on and REM-off neurons in the mesopontine tegmentum underlie a bistable flip–flop mechanism regulating REM sleep onset and termination by means of sequential mutual inhibition. The area of GABAergic REM-on neurons contains also glutamatergic neurons projecting either to the basal forebrain to produce, together with the activation of the cholinergic system, the EEG desynchronisation or to the medulla to activate neurons eliciting the inhibition of spinal motoneurons underlying the skeletal muscle atonia typical of REM sleep. Glycine is the neurotransmitter of such tonic inhibition that is irregularly masked by brief excitatory influences producing twitches and jerks, usually during periods of rapid eye movements (see Chase and Morales, 2005). Also the almost immediate restoring of homeostatic responses to thermal loads on arousal from REM sleep demonstrates the existence of an inverse poikilostasis–homeostasis switch, depending on GABAergic REM-off neurons of the bistable flip–flop mechanism. Another mechanism underlying REM sleep onset has been suggested that connects the hypothalamus with the REM sleep-inducing structures in the pons (Fort *et al.*, 2009). It is based on the activation of GABAergic neurones located in the posterior hypothalamus, ventrolateral periaqueductal gray and dorsal pontine paragigantocellular reticular nucleus in association with the drop in activity of the orexinergic/hypocretinergic excitatory system of the lateral hypothalamus active in wakefulness. GABAergic inhibition also brings about the suppression of the inhibition of glutamatergic neurons exciting the neurons exerting the glycinergic inhibition of spinal motoneurons underlying skeletal muscle atonia in REM sleep. The end of REM sleep depends on the inhibition of the previous GABAergic inhibition by activation of GABAergic neurons of the ventrolateral periaqueductal gray, together with pontine and medullary noradrenergic and hypothalamic orexinergic/hypocretinergic neurons.

Besides the control of REM sleep occurrence, the physiological effects of such switch mechanisms differ according to the function and the species considered. If the function is strictly controlled by an imperative diencephalic command, REM sleep is characterised by the suppression of this specific homeostatic control (e.g., thermoregulation). If the function is controlled by a set of potentially autonomous but hierarchically coordinated mechanisms, distributed along the hypothalamic-mesencephalic-pontomedullar axis of the central nervous system, impairment of precise homeostatic control but not of the basic function itself is observed (e.g., circulation and respiration in cats, rabbits, rats, humans). In other words, the functional controls requiring high hierarchical levels of integration are the most affected during REM sleep, whereas reflex activity is only altered but not obliterated. In the latter case, the changes depend on a deficient homeostatic modulation of reflexes by the modified central command in REM sleep. On the whole, the study of physiological operators is a reliable tool to infer indirectly sleep-dependent changes in the neural control of homeostasis.

Perspective

The operational definition of the principle of homeostasis may appear conceptually simple in theory. The previous discussions, however, show that its definition is much more demanding and complex in practice.

The study of the principle of homeostasis is here limited to the realm of physiological functions in terrestrial species. Whatever the difficulty of moving across such different physiological processes may be, it is clear, however *a posteriori*, that from the evolutionary viewpoint the change from a homeostatic to a poikilostatic regulation modality in REM sleep does not entail a life threat under normal circumstances. Nevertheless, in mammals, whatever the evolutionary path, NREM sleep and particularly REM sleep always raises problems for physiological regulation. A regulation that ought to be consistent with the ecosystem in which they live. This is quite apparent in sea mammals. Slow waves of NREM sleep occur in only one brain hemisphere at a time (unihemispheric sleep), while the awake hemisphere controls breathing and engagement with the environment (Mukhametov *et al.*, 1985). Rather than a total absence of REM sleep, which is a dangerous event for breathing species living in water, there is probably an extreme shortening of the episodes and a small number of them. This is true in cases in which they are identified only by phasic events, like twitches and jerks. The result is a remarkably short total daily duration of REM sleep with respect to terrestrial mammals (see Zepelin *et al.*, 2005; Siegel, 2005). The species-specific differences in the ultradian and circadian expression, as well as the physiological regulation of REM sleep, therefore, leave many questions unanswered concerning the functional significance of this behavioural state.

The methodological criteria presented in this and the previous chapter underlie the approach to follow regarding the physiological issues addressed in the book. The presentation is far from being complete but is hopefully sufficient. The vast store of literature is presented mainly in relation to the issue of homeostasis in order to avoid overburdening the reader. In addition to this relative restraint, it is also important to inform the reader that the majority of the experimental results discussed were obtained from representatives of three orders of the mammalian class, namely cat (Carnivora), rabbit (Lagomorpha) and rat (Rodentia). The experimental study in human homeostasis during sleep was not as radical and complete as in animals since it was kept under reasonably restrained experimental conditions. Nevertheless, the contribution of sleep medicine to sleep physiology and pathology in humans has brought about fundamental observations concerning the issue of homeostasis particularly in the realm of respiration and circulation, as is shown by the list of references.

The modulation in sleep of gastrointestinal and renal functions is not considered in this book since it does not fit within the strict temporal criterion of the homeostasis–poikilostasis dichotomy in the ultradian cycle of sleep. In addition, the sleep-state-dependent changes in the secretion of somatotropin, prolactine, thyrotropin, gonadotropins and the hormones underlying the hydromineral balance, cannot be simply considered the result of the alternation between homeostasis and poikilostasis. The secretion of these physiological operators appears to be modulated across the ultradian sleep cycle for long-term physiological processes, such as growth, basal metabolic rate and sexual cycle, and not only as a result of the short-lasting deficit of homeostatic regulation in REM sleep. In particular, concerning the control of the osmolality of extracellular fluid, it has been shown that the antidiuretic response to osmotic stimulation of the magnocellular neurons of the hypothalamic paraventricular and supraoptic nuclei is not significantly affected during REM sleep (Luppi *et al.*, 2010). In this respect, a study of the influence of sleep states on thyrotropin release under thermal loads would help delimit further the physiological boundaries of the homeostasis–poikilostasis dichotomy in sleep.

Conclusion

The manner of introducing next the systemic physiological functions examined in this book, namely respiration, circulation and thermoregulation, deserves a preliminary comment to avoid, perhaps, a conceptual misunderstanding concerning the order and the different elaborations of their presentation.

Respiration and circulation are approached first in the next two chapters because they have primary and associated roles in the general process of maintaining the homeostasis of all tissues of the body. The general importance of the combination of both functions for the control of the physical and chemical processes of cellular life is self-evident. Actually, the two functions cannot independently operate in the living organism. They may be considered as systemic operators, that together directly support the homeostasis of all the vital physiological parameters. Respiratory and circulatory failures independently or together produce life-threatening changes in the controlled physiological parameters in much shorter time than in the case of the alteration of other physiological functions, including thermoregulation. However, respiration and circulation are separately considered in order to simplify the presentation of the experimental results that bear upon the problem under study. Such subdivision of roles is conceptually more tractable.

The presentation of data in the following chapters dealing with the homeostasis of respiration, circulation and thermoregulation in sleep is not uniform as far as extension and depth of the arguments are concerned. Such differences do not depend on the functional criterion of their immediate importance with respect to the survival of the organism. The analysis of homeostasis is based, instead, on the axiom that the development of the sophisticated mechanisms for the neural control of temperature in mammals required also an adequate implementation of the pre-existing functions of respiration and circulation and not vice versa. This conceptual order only stresses the biological importance of losing the self-control of temperature by the mammalian organism during REM sleep.

The appropriation of a universal physical variable as an internal physiological parameter for a precise non-specific regulation (optimisation) of the physical and chemical processes of the organism was an important evolutionary event. A thermal condition that, however, requires a most accurate neural control of its homeostasis. A control that is especially demanding because temperature is a variable that cannot be easily maintained stationary in value and conveniently compartmentalised in different parts of the body without energy expenditure for active and passive defence of homeothermy. Thermoregulation in mammals is, therefore, the most impressive functional expression of the principle of homeostasis and the direct evidence of the control exerted by the central nervous system over the interaction between internal and external environment.

Chapter 3

Respiration in Sleep

Respiration consists of the exchange of O_2 and CO_2 between body tissues and the environment as result of lung ventilation and blood circulation. Basically, there are automatic and behavioural control mechanisms of respiration. The neurons of the automatic generator of breathing are located in the medulla and pons and are influenced by specific inputs of mechano- and chemoceptive feedback loops. Also, other neuronal networks interact with ponto-medullary and spinal respiratory neurons according to a variety of behavioural functional requests. The behavioural control modulates breathing according to physiological needs during wakefulness. Behavioural control includes reflex (e.g., coughing, sneezing, muscle exercise ventilation, etc.), thermoregulatory (tachypnea and panting in some mammalian species) and voluntary (e.g., ventilation during muscular exercise, phonation) mechanisms that are distributed at different levels of the neuraxis.

From the functional viewpoint, changes in breathing characterise each state of sleep compared with wakefulness. In the condition of normal health, the homeostasis–poikilostasis switch of the central integrative command during the ultradian sleep cycle remarkably affects the automatic ventilation rhythm that underlies the basic respiratory function of gas exchange. Before providing a more detailed description of the effects of this switching, the general changes of breathing during the sleep states are briefly summarised.

In NREM sleep, a reversible release of breathing from the behavioural control in wakefulness sets in, but the automatic control remains operative. In REM sleep, a conflicting interaction develops between automatic and behavioural controls that makes the animal prone to disturbances in breathing. Data demonstrating the physiological expression of the significant changes occurring in the regulation of breathing during the behavioural states of sleep are documented below. They reveal that the functional dichotomy between NREM sleep and REM sleep in terms of homeostatic and poikilostatic control, respectively, is a characteristic feature not only of thermoregulation but also of the respiratory function.

Control of Respiration in Sleep

In the transition from wakefulness to NREM sleep the automatic control mechanism is released from the behavioural influence of wakefulness (Fink, 1961; Lydic and Orem, 1979; Mitchell and Berger, 1975; Netick and Foutz, 1980; Orem, 1980; Orem *et al.*, 1974, 1977b; Phillipson, 1977; Phillipson *et al.*, 1976a). This transition (stages I and II of NREM sleep in humans) is characterised by breathing instability (Duron, 1972; Gillam, 1972; Reite *et al.*, 1975; Snyder *et al.*, 1964; Specht and Fruhmann, 1972; Trinder *et al.*, 1992; Tusiewicz *et al.*, 1977; Webb and Hiestand, 1975) and the appearance of respiratory and circulatory periodic phenomena (Bülow, 1963; Duron, 1972; Lugaresi *et al.*, 1972) that may be considered as release phenomena underlying the development of a new functional equilibrium in the automatic control of breathing.

NREM Sleep

After this functional transition, regular breathing sets in with deep NREM sleep (stages III and IV in humans) when breathing is driven by the automatic control mechanism alone. The breathing rate decreases and the tidal volume increases slightly with the result that ventilation decreases in humans (Birchfield *et al.*, 1959; Bülow, 1963; Bülow and Ingvar, 1961) and animals (Orem *et al.*, 1977b; Phillipson *et al.*, 1976a) due to the decrease in metabolic rate. An increase in alveolar CO_2 partial pressure in humans (Bülow, 1963; Bülow and Ingvar, 1961) and animals (Phillipson, 1977; Phillipson and Bowes, 1986), and in arterial CO_2 partial pressure in humans (Birchfield *et al.*, 1958, 1959) and cats (Guazzi and Freis, 1969) have been observed. These changes are associated with a decrease in alveolar and arterial O_2 partial pressure in humans (Robin *et al.*, 1958) and cats (Guazzi and Freis, 1969). Airway resistance is increased (Orem *et al.*, 1977a; Robin *et al.*, 1958).

These changes in the physiological operators of respiration are consistent with a state of rest requiring lower energy expenditure than in wakefulness. Although the operation of the automatic control mechanism appears to be down-regulated, the physiological responses underlying respiratory homeostasis are normally elicited in NREM sleep. Respiratory chemosensitivity to CO_2 is only moderately reduced (Bellville *et al.*, 1959; Birchfield *et al.*, 1959; Bülow, 1963; Reed and Kellogg, 1958; Robin *et al.*, 1958). The respiratory response to hypoxia is, however, unaffected in humans (Reed and Kellogg, 1960) and in the dog (Phillipson *et al.*, 1978). Moreover, pulmonary inflation and deflation reflexes are active during NREM sleep both in human infants (Finer *et al.*, 1976) and animals (Farber and Marlow, 1976; Phillipson *et al.*, 1976a). The responses to a mechanical respiratory load (airway occlusion, inspiration from a rigid container increasing breathing work) are also practically identical to those observed during wakefulness (Phillipson *et al.*, 1976b), thus showing that the proprioceptive reflexes of the intercostal muscles are normal during NREM sleep.

REM Sleep

The physiological phenomena of REM sleep show a marked alteration in the activity of the automatic control mechanism of breathing. What follows is a description of phenomena observed in various species. It is clear that not mentioning all species for many of the phenomena does not imply that the results would not be the same if studied in that species unless there may be species-specific phenomena. The respiratory rhythm in humans and animals is irregular (Aserinsky, 1965; Aserinsky and Kleitman, 1953; Duron, 1972; Phillipson, 1978; Snyder *et al.*, 1964). The average frequency is increased or decreased in cats with respect to the rate attained during NREM sleep in eupnea or polypnea respectively (Parmeggiani, 1978, 1979; Parmeggiani and Sabattini, 1972). The respiratory activity of the intercostal muscles is diminished in cats (Fig. 3) and lambs (Duron, 1969; Henderson-Smart and Read, 1978; Islas-Marroquin, 1966; Parmeggiani and Sabattini, 1972; Parmeggiani *et al.*, 1973). In human infants this depression may even produce paradoxical chest collapse during inspiration (Tusiewicz *et al.*, 1977). Ventilation increases in humans (Bolton and Herman, 1974; Bülow, 1963; Fagenholz *et al.*, 1976; Finer *et al.*, 1976; Hathorn, 1974; Purcell,

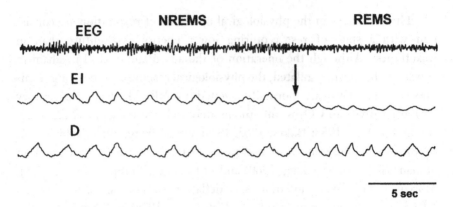

Fig. 3. Spontaneous immediate depression of the activity of respiratory muscles at the transition from NREMS to REMS (cat). The integrated electromyogram of the respiratory bursts of the external intercostal muscles (EI) drops markedly in magnitude at REMS onset (arrow), whereas that of the diaphragm (D) is not significantly affected in amplitude. EEG, electroencephalogram; NREMS, NREM sleep; REMS, REM sleep. (Modified from Parmeggiani *et al.*, 1973.)

1976) and dogs (Phillipson *et al.*, 1977), mostly in temporal relation to myoclonic twitches (Orem *et al.*, 1977b; Wurtz and O'Flaerty, 1967). Alveolar ventilation is variable as shown either by a decrease (Bülow, 1963; Phillipson *et al.*, 1976a; Wurtz and O'Flaerty, 1967) or no change (Fagenholz *et al.*, 1976; Guazzi and Freis, 1969; Remmers *et al.*, 1976) in alveolar CO_2 partial pressure. Upper airway resistance increases in humans and cats (Henke *et al.*, 1991; Orem *et al.*, 1977a; Wiegand *et al.*, 1991). The compensation of a respiratory load is irregular and weak in humans (Frantz *et al.*, 1976; Henke *et al.*, 1992; Knill *et al.*, 1976; Purcell, 1976) and lambs (Henderson-Smart and Read, 1978). Such disturbances appear to depend on the influence of telencephalic and diencephalic behavioural commands. This is shown by the following experimental results. The disturbances persist after vagotomy (Dawes *et al.*, 1972; Phillipson *et al.*, 1976a; Remmers *et al.*, 1976), sectioning of the spinal cord at T_{1-2} (Puizillout *et al.*, 1974; Thach *et al.*, 1977), afferent denervation of the mid-thoracic chest wall (Phillipson, 1977), denervation of the carotid and aortic chemo- and baroreceptors (Guazzi and Freis, 1969), in hypercapnia (Phillipson *et al.*, 1977) and hypoxia (Phillipson *et al.*, 1978).

Other phenomena accompany the alteration of the automatic control mechanism of breathing during REM sleep. The response to hypercapnia is further depressed with respect to NREM sleep in adult humans (Berthon-Jones and Sullivan, 1984; Douglas *et al.*, 1982; White, 1986) and adult dogs and cats (Bryan *et al.*, 1976; Netick *et al.*, 1984; Phillipson *et al.*, 1977; Santiago *et al.*, 1981; Sullivan *et al.*, 1979). The response to hypoxia in adult animals is either unchanged (Bolton and Herman, 1974; Fagenholz *et al.*, 1976; Phillipson *et al.*, 1978) or depressed (Bowes *et al.*, 1981; Santiago *et al.*, 1984), whereas it is depressed with respect to NREM sleep in adult humans (Berthon-Jones and Sullivan, 1982; Douglas *et al.*, 1982; Hedemark and Kronenberg, 1982). The inflation reflex is practically abolished during REM sleep in dogs (Phillipson *et al.*, 1976a) and human infants (Finer *et al.*, 1976). Although the pulmonary deflation and inflation reflexes persist in the opossum, they are more variable in REM sleep than during NREM sleep (Farber and Marlow, 1976). Table 1 presents general functional differences between NREM sleep and REM sleep.

Central Command of Breathing in Sleep

The brain's control of breathing is remarkably depressed during REM sleep as compared to NREM sleep. This is shown in cats by the disappearance in REM sleep of the tachypnea elicited by means of direct thermal

Table 1. General changes in respiration across the ultradian sleep states.

Respiration	NREMS versus Q. WAKE	REMS versus NREMS
Breathing rate	Decreased	Variable
Tidal volume	Increased	Variable
Ventilation	Decreased	Variable
Inflation reflex	Normal	Depressed
Deflation reflex	Normal	Depressed
Proprioceptive reflexes	Normal	Depressed
Alveolar pCO_2	Increased	Variable
Alveolar pO_2	Decreased	Variable

Note: Functional stability and normal reflex control of respiration in NREMS in contrast with functional variability and reflex depression in REMS. Q. WAKE, quiet wakefulness; NREMS, NREM sleep; REMS, REM sleep.

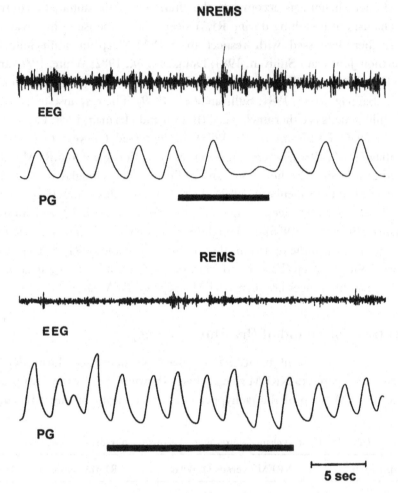

Fig. 4. Respiratory effects of repetitive electrical stimulation of the preoptic-anterior hypo-thalamic area during sleep (cat). Lung inflation-like effect elicited by stimulation in NREMS (0.13 mA, 5 msec, 10/sec). Increased intensity and duration of stimulation is ineffective in REMS (0.15 mA, 5 msec, 10/sec). EEG, electroencephalogram; PG, pneumogram; NREMS, NREM sleep; REMS, REM sleep. (Modified from Parmeggiani *et al.*, 1981.)

stimulation of the preoptic-anterior hypothalamic area in the thermoneu-tral zone of ambient temperature (Parmeggiani *et al.*, 1973, 1976). The effect of warming during NREM sleep persists after the end of stimulation as long as the preoptic-anterior hypothalamic temperature is higher than the threshold temperature of tachypnea. The tachypnea elicited by preoptic-anterior hypothalamic warming during NREM sleep immediately disappears with the advent of an episode of REM sleep even though the preoptic-anterior hypothalamic temperature is still above the NREM sleep threshold of the respiratory response. Also preoptic-anterior hypothalamic warming of higher intensity than that delivered during NREM sleep elicits no significant respiratory response during REM sleep. On awakening, tachypnea appears immediately if preoptic-anterior hypothalamic temperature is still above threshold.

The lung inflation- or deflation-like responses elicited by direct electrical stimulation of the preoptic-anterior hypothalamic area are suppressed during REM sleep (Parmeggiani *et al.*, 1981) (Fig. 4). Moreover, electrical stimulation of the orbital frontal cortex in cats produces respiratory phase switching during quiet waking and NREM sleep but not during REM sleep (Marks *et al.*, 1987).

Conclusion

A complete and detailed study of the functional relationships of all the physiological parameters and operators presented in this chapter is beyond the scope of this book. The general conclusion is already warranted that the physiological features of NREM sleep and REM sleep are consistent and inconsistent, respectively, with the principle of homeostasis.

The down-regulation of breathing in NREM sleep is physiologically consistent with the predictive homeostasis of a state of motor and postural quiescence and lower metabolic rate with respect to wakefulness. Moreover, the feedback controls of reactive homeostasis are still operative. In other words, the functional changes in breathing are in full agreement with the behavioural quiescence of NREM sleep. They depend on a specific setting of the homeostatic control of respiration by the preoptic-anterior hypothalamic area in the absence of telencephalic behavioural commands. In contrast, the experimental evidence demonstrates that in passing from NREM sleep to REM sleep a homeostasis-poikilostasis switch occurs in the control of breathing. In REM sleep there is a remarkable instability and depression of the respiratory operators as a result of variable and conflicting telencephalic and diencephalic behavioural commands on the pontomedullary neuronal networks and the reflex mechanisms of breathing.

Chapter 4

Circulation in Sleep

The study of circulation in sleep from the viewpoint of homeostasis is more complex than that of respiration and thermoregulation. The homeostatic function of circulation does not have a selective, direct target of just a few physiological parameters (O_2, CO_2, H^+) or of a single physiological parameter (temperature) as in the case of respiration and thermoregulation, respectively. Circulation is fundamentally, although only indirectly, implicated in the maintenance of the homeostasis of all the physiological parameters of the organism. This result depends on the cardiovascular operators underlying the dynamic distribution of the blood to the different body tissues.

Control of Circulation

The circulation of blood is controlled by a regulatory system that presents multiple operative levels of increasing integrative complexity. Peripheral flow–metabolism coupling and vascular auto-regulation, spinal and rhombencephalic autonomic reflex mechanisms and diencephalic–telencephalic integrative commands are the principal operative levels of this distributed regulatory system.

The study of cardiovascular regulation across the states of the ultradian sleep cycle has shown that NREM sleep and REM sleep are basically different behavioural states, being broadly characterised by coordinated and uncoordinated changes in cardiovascular operators, respectively. The systematic comparison of the changes in the variables on passing from NREM sleep to REM sleep clearly shows the effect of the homeostasis–poikilostasis switch in circulatory regulation.

During NREM sleep, the cardiovascular phenomena are, in general, consistent with the reduced metabolic demand of behavioural rest: the suspension of goal-directed motor and postural activity. In contrast, the homeostatic inconsistency of REM sleep is marked by autogenously variable control of the activity of cardiovascular operators. Nevertheless, the changes observed in the circulatory function during REM sleep are never as radical as the full suspension of the thermoregulatory function. The reason for this difference is that the control of the effectors of many thermoregulatory responses, which also involve the respiratory and circulatory functions, is centralised in the preoptic-hypothalamic area, particularly in furry species. In contrast, in all species studied the vital controls of physiological operators underlying blood circulation are organised not only at brain stem and spinal levels but also peripherally at heart and tissue levels (e.g., auto-regulation of heart muscle contractility and of capillary blood flow). In normal conditions, the central instability of cardiovascular regulation in REM sleep does not impair the essential blood supply to body tissues, and particularly the heart and the brain (see Chapter 7).

Changes of Circulation in Sleep

The next part of this chapter presents a sample of the typical circulatory features of sleep that support the previous conclusions. The most studied cardiovascular operators of different orders of complexity are heart rate (Fig. 5), stroke volume, cardiac output, regional vascular conductance, arterial blood pressure, baroreceptive and chemoreceptive reflexes.

NREM Sleep

The coordinated down-regulation of cardiovascular functions during NREM sleep is fully consistent with the quiescent behavioural state in the mammalian species studied. From a general viewpoint, the agreement of experimental results with the principle of homeostasis across several decades of research is noteworthy. The presentation of experimental data that follows compares the functional changes in NREM sleep in relation to

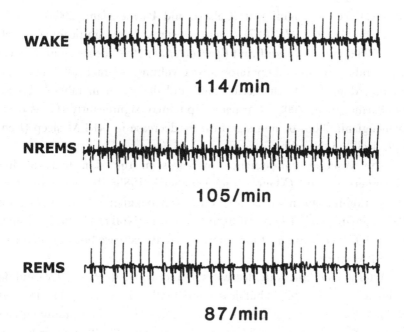

WAKE

114/min

NREMS

105/min

REMS

87/min

Fig. 5. Changes in the spontaneous heart rate (EKG) during wake–sleep states (cat). The heart rate is regular in wakefulness and decreases in NREMS, whereas a marked brad-yarrhythmia characterises REMS. Wake, wakefulness; NREMS, NREM sleep; REMS, REM sleep. (Modified from Azzaroni and Parmeggiani, 1993.)

those of quiet wakefulness. It is likely that the small quantitative variability (i.e., between invariance and slight decrease) of cardiovascular operators observed during NREM sleep with respect to quiet wakefulness among species and within species described below depends on the pre-existing activity levels in waking as a result of the unnatural experimental conditions. In addition, the differences in statistical significance may also depend on the different techniques used for such measurements (e.g., radioactive microspheres or flowmeters).

Of the cardiac operators influencing cardiac output, namely, heart rate and stroke volume, the first is moderately decreased in human subjects (Bristow *et al.*, 1969; Iellamo *et al.*, 2004; Khatri and Freis, 1967; Snyder *et al.*, 1964; Somers *et al.*, 1993; van de Borne *et al.*, 1994), dogs (Schneider *et al.*, 1997), cats (Baust and Bohnert, 1969; Mancia and Zanchetti, 1980) and mice (Schaub *et al.*, 1998). In rabbits the decrease is statistically either significant (Calasso and Parmeggiani, 2008) or non-significant (Lenzi *et al.*, 1987). There is a statistically significant (Lacombe *et al.*, 1988) and non-significant (Zoccoli *et al.*, 1994) decrease in the heart rate of rats. The second operator, stroke volume, is practically unchanged in cats (Mancia and Zanchetti, 1980) and decreased in rabbits (Calasso and Parmeggiani, 2008). Cardiac output may significantly (Calasso and Parmeggiani, 2008) or non-significantly decrease in NREM sleep (Lenzi *et al.*, 1987) in the rabbit.

The vascular conductance increases in the skin beds of heat exchangers in cats (Mancia and Zanchetti, 1980; Parmeggiani *et al.*, 1977), rabbits (Franzini *et al.*, 1982; Parmeggiani *et al.*, 1998), rats (Parmeggiani *et al.*, 1998) and human subjects (Noll *et al.*, 1994; Sindrup *et al.*, 1992), creating heat loss increases that decrease body temperature in NREM sleep.

Arterial blood pressure decreases in mice (Schaub *et al.*, 1998) and dog (Schneider *et al.*, 1997), but less consistently in the cat (Mancia *et al.*, 1971), rabbit (Cianci *et al.*, 1991; Lenzi *et al.*, 1987) and rat (Junqueira and Krieger, 1976; Lacombe *et al.*, 1988; Meunier *et al.*, 1988; Zoccoli *et al.*, 1994). Tonic decrease in arterial blood pressure has also been observed in human subjects (Carrington *et al.*, 2005; Coccagna *et al.*, 1971; Iellamo *et al.*, 2004; Jones *et al.*, 1982; Khatri and Freis, 1967; Monti *et al.*, 2002; Scharf, 1984; Snyder *et al.*, 1964; Somers *et al.*, 1993; Tank *et al.*, 2003; van de Borne *et al.*, 1994), although intensity varied depending on the subject (Mancia, 1993). Further, less variability of arterial blood pressure in NREM sleep than in wakefulness has been demonstrated in human subjects (Monti *et al.*, 2002; van de Borne *et al.*, 1994) and rats (Lacombe *et al.*, 1988; Silvani *et al.*, 2003).

Finally, the baroreflex control of vasculature and heart rhythm is still effective during NREM sleep in human subjects (see Silvani and Lenzi, 2005). In cats (Del Bo *et al.*, 1985), lambs (Horne *et al.*, 1991) and rats (Nagura *et al.*, 2004; Zoccoli *et al.*, 2001), the baroreflex gain (response to stimulus ratio) shows no substantial difference with respect to wakefulness. Muscle sympathetic nerve activity decreases in humans (Somers *et al.*, 1993) and renal sympathetic nerve activity in rats correlates positively with the decreased arterial pressure (Miki *et al.*, 2003). The baroreflex gain in renal (Combs *et al.*, 1986) and in muscle (Nakazato *et al.*, 1998) sympathetic nerves in baboons and humans, respectively, is lower in NREM sleep than in wakefulness according to the general decrease in sympathetic activity during this state of sleep.

On the whole, the changes observed in cardiovascular operators in all the species studied during NREM sleep appear either statistically non-significant or tending to a rather uniform quantitative decrease with respect to quiet wakefulness. They are also consistent with the principle of physiological homeostasis in a condition of motor and postural quiescence that is characterised by a controlled decrease in body temperature and in the energy demand with respect to wakefulness.

REM Sleep

Much greater qualitative and quantitative variability of physiological phenomena characterises REM sleep within and between species compared to NREM sleep. The difference of REM sleep from NREM sleep is also related to the intrinsical variability of the former as a result of the phasic and tonic periods of the state. Phasic REM sleep presents muscle twitching and bursts of rapid-eye-movements that lack in tonic REM sleep. Variability may be considered the fundamental feature of the poikilostatic neural regulation of REM sleep. The best reason for this conclusion is that the same species and experimental conditions are also inherent in the experimental study of NREM sleep. This state is characterised by uniformity rather than variability of the observed physiological phenomena among and within species.

Heart rate in human subjects may (Khatri and Freis, 1967; Snyder *et al.*, 1964; Somers *et al.*, 1993; van de Borne *et al.*, 1994) or may not (Iellamo *et al.*, 2004; Monti *et al.*, 2002) increase. A decrease in heart rate was observed in cats early after surgery (Mancia *et al.*, 1971) and an increase after a prolonged recovery from surgery (Sei *et al.*, 1989). In rats, an increase (Sei and Morita, 1996b; Sei *et al.*, 2002), a decrease (Miki *et al.*, 2003, 2004; Nagura *et al.*, 2004; Yoshimoto *et al.*, 2004) and a non–significant change (Lacombe *et al.*, 1988; Zoccoli *et al.*, 2001) in heart rate were reported. In rabbits (Fig. 6), heart rate (bradyarrhythmia), stroke volume

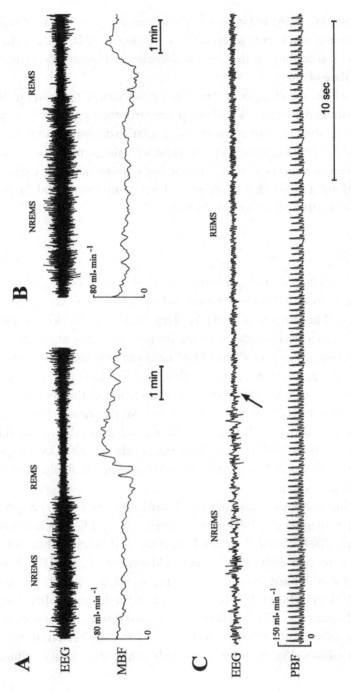

Fig. 6.   Changes in common carotid blood flow during sleep (rabbit). A and B: mean blood flow (MBF) decreases with increasing negative slope from NREMS to REMS. C: peak blood flow (PBF) decreases to a minimum in REMS that is also characterised by marked brady-arrhythmia. EEG, electroencephalogram; NREMS, NREM sleep; REMS, REM sleep. (Modified from Calasso and Parmeggiani, 2008.)

and cardiac output decreased significantly in a study using the flowmeter (Calasso and Parmeggiani, 2008), and non-significantly in another study using microspheres for flow determination (Lenzi *et al.*, 1987).

The arterial pressure increases in human subjects (Coccagna *et al.*, 1971; Iellamo *et al.*, 2004; Khatri and Freis, 1967; Somers *et al.*, 1993; van de Borne *et al.*, 1994), rats (Junqueira and Krieger, 1976; Miki *et al.*, 2003, 2004; Nagura *et al.*, 2004; Sei *et al.*, 1999; Yoshimoto *et al.*, 2004) and rabbits (Cianci *et al.*, 1991). Arterial pressure decreases in dogs (Schneider *et al.*, 1997) and pigs (Zinkovska *et al.*, 1996). A decrease had been described in cats (Baccelli *et al.*, 1974; Gassel *et al.*, 1964; Guazzi *et al.*, 1968; Kumazawa *et al.*, 1969; Mancia *et al.*, 1971), but later experiments revealed that pressure also increases if more post-operative time is allowed (Sei *et al.*, 1989, 1994). In this respect, it is not clear whether, besides recovery from surgery, the influence of stress due to prolongation of the experiment may also play a role. Also the ambient temperature influencing the vasomotion of heat exchangers (Sei and Morita, 1996a) complicates the results of the experimental study of arterial pressure control in REM sleep (see Silvani, 2008).

A striking feature of REM sleep in different species is the fluctuation of arterial blood pressure and heart rate. Fluctuation occurs in all species studied: rats (Berteotti *et al.*, 2008; Junqueira and Krieger, 1976; Sei and Morita, 1996b), cats (Gassel *et al.*, 1964; Guazzi and Zanchetti, 1965; Mancia *et al.*, 1971), rabbits (Dufour and Court, 1977), mice (Campen *et al.*, 2002), lambs (Fewell, 1993) and humans (Coccagna *et al.*, 1971; Jones *et al.*, 1982; Scharf, 1984; Snyder *et al.*, 1964; Somers *et al.*, 1993). They are in general loosely associated with bursts of rapid eye movements, myoclonic twitches and, probably more often, breathing irregularities.

Arterial blood pressure may fall in cats as a result of a pronounced bradycardia associated with a practically unchanged stroke volume and an increase in total vascular conductance: the increase in vascular conductance in the skin, mesenteric and renal beds prevails over the decrease in conductance of the hindlimb muscle vasculature (Baccelli *et al.*, 1974; Mancia and Zanchetti, 1980). In the rabbit, renal and fat vascular conductance appears to be decreased during REM sleep (Lenzi *et al.*, 1987). The poor correlation between regional and systemic variables shows that the central integration of cardiovascular functions is altered in REM sleep.

In cats, arterial blood pressure during REM sleep is still buffered by sinoaortic reflexes (Guazzi and Zanchetti, 1965; Iwamura *et al.*, 1969). After sinoaortic denervation, arterial blood pressure is mildly increased during wakefulness, decreases to slightly more than that which occurs in normal animals during NREM sleep and then decreases sharply during REM sleep. This decrease in some REM episodes may produce brain ischemia as revealed by a flattening of the electroencephalogram, motor convulsions and arousal (Guazzi and Zanchetti, 1965). The drop of arterial blood pressure after sinoaortic denervation depends on the greater vasodilation in the splanchnic vascular bed and the reversal of vasoconstriction to vasodilation in the hindlimb muscles (Baccelli *et al.*, 1978; Mancia and Zanchetti, 1980). Selective removal of either baroreceptor or chemoreceptor afferents showed that the arterial hypotension of REM sleep is buffered in the cat primarily by chemoreceptor reflexes because baroreceptor reflexes are depressed in this species (Guazzi *et al.*, 1968; Knuepfer *et al.*, 1986; Mancia and Zanchetti, 1980). In the rat, arterial blood pressure increases during REM sleep, whereas in sinoaortic-denervated rats hypotension (Junqueira and Krieger, 1976) or hypertension (Sei *et al.*, 1999) was observed. The role of baroreceptors in REM sleep is still problematic also because enough time may not have been allowed for post-operative recovery (Sei *et al.*, 1994). Also, the results of baroreceptor studies in humans suggest caution in this respect because reflex sensitivity may either increase (Jones *et al.*, 1982) or decrease (Conway *et al.*, 1983) in REM sleep. At this point, it appears likely that circulation in different species is affected by similar central influences in REM sleep, although the eventual pattern of change in cardiovascular variables also depends on species-specific differences in the operation of feedback loops (Gilmore and Tomomatsu, 1984) and peripheral auto-regulation (Cowley *et al.*, 1989).

In conclusion, the actual cardiac output is the result of a poor correlation between heart rate, stroke volume and arterial blood pressure, associated with tonic and phasic changes in vascular conductance. All this underlies the apparently meaningless changes in the regional distribution of cardiac output with respect to NREM sleep (Cianci *et al.*, 1991). A good example of altered vasomotion in REM is the fact that sleep vasodilatation of heat exchangers occurs in the cold, while, vasoconstriction occurs in warm conditions, both in cats (Parmeggiani *et al.*, 1977) and rabbits (Franzini *et al.*, 1982), as mentioned in Chapter 5.

The variability of cardiovascular phenomena is not simply the direct result of changes in the central regulation of the autonomic outflow; it is also loosely associated with bursts of rapid eye movements, myoclonic twitches, ponto-geniculo-occipital waves and breathing irregularities. These centrally driven influences also indirectly activate a number of feedback loops by affecting the peripherally controlled physiological parameters (Baust and Bohnert, 1969; Gassel *et al.*, 1964). During REM sleep, therefore, the interaction between the variable influences of the central commands and the variable feedback information from the periphery, that may influence reflex responses, is a further factor in the generation of REM sleep instability of cardiovascular regulation (see Parmeggiani, 1994). The importance of such an interaction is also shown by studies in anesthetised (Gebber *et al.*, 1990) and awake (Ninomiya *et al.*, 1990) cats, which demonstrated that the central generator underlying the rhythmicity of synchronised cardiac sympathetic nerve activity is subject to reflex modulation by baroreceptor inputs. In addition, the patterns of change in cardiovascular variables also depend on species-specific differences in the operation of feedback loops (Gilmore and Tomomatsu, 1984; Sindrup *et al.*, 1992) and auto-regulation (Baccelli *et al.*, 1974; Cowley *et al.*, 1989). However, the prevalence of an unstable central autonomic command plays a substantial role in the variability of circulatory events in REM sleep (see Parmeggiani, 1994; Silvani and Lenzi, 2005). Table 2 presents general functional differences between NREM sleep and REM sleep.

Central Command of Circulation in Sleep

Concerning the control of the brain integrative centres on cardiovascular regulation (Behbehani and Da Costa, 1996; Hirasawa *et al.*, 1996; Hosoya *et al.*, 1991; Kanosue *et al.*, 1994a), experimental data reveal that thermoregulatory vasomotion (pinna of the ear) elicited by direct thermal stimulation of the preoptic-anterior hypothalamic region during NREM sleep is suppressed during REM sleep in cats (Fig. 8, Chapter 5) (Parmeggiani *et al.*, 1977). This result is in agreement with the reduced responsiveness of preoptic-hypothalamic thermosensitive neurons (Alam *et al.*, 1995a,b; Glotzbach and Heller, 1984; Parmeggiani *et al.*, 1983, 1986, 1987). Moreover, a depression of the amygdala control over cardiovascular activity has been observed in cats during REM sleep (Frysinger *et al.*, 1984).

Table 2. General changes in circulation across the ultradian sleep states.

Circulation	NREMS versus Q. WAKE	REMS versus NREMS
Heart rate	Decreased	Variable
Stroke volume	Decreased	Variable
Cardiac output	Decreased	Variable
Vascular conductance	Increased	Variable
Blood pressure	Decreased	Variable
Baroreflex	Normal	Variable
Chemoreflex	Normal	Variable

Note: Functional stability and normal reflex control of circulation in NREMS in contrast with functional variability and reflex instability in REMS. Q. WAKE, quiet wakefulness; NREMS, NREM sleep; REMS, REM sleep.

Electrical stimulation of the region of the central nucleus of the amygdala during waking and sleep states elicited a pressor response. The response was attenuated in NREM sleep and greatly depressed in REM sleep. According to the authors, REM sleep involves a functional dissociation between forebrain and brain stem systems underlying cardiovascular regulation.

Conclusion

Like the changes observed in the activity of the respiratory operators, those of the cardiovascular operators are consistent with the somatic motor quiescence and reduced metabolic rate of NREM sleep. Equally consistent are the increase in the parasympathetic and decrease in the sympathetic influence on the heart. In contrast, a change in the central integration of cardiovascular operators in REM sleep brings about uncoordinated and irregular cardiovascular phenomena.

The conclusion is that the cardiovascular activity in NREM sleep fits in well with the harmonic somatic and autonomic functional expression of a homeostatic state. In contrast, all the experimental data show that the integrative, homeostatic control of cardiovascular operators is disrupted sufficiently in REM sleep to qualify it as poikilostatic from the viewpoint of physiological regulation.

Chapter 5

Temperature Regulation in Sleep

The control of body temperature is the clearest example of homeostatic regulation in mammals. The underlying mechanisms are complex, consisting of activity in several physiological functions, somatic and autonomic, both under the integrative control of the central nervous system.

In this chapter, body temperature will be first considered in general. Then, the contribution to thermoregulation in sleep of the motor and postural activity of skeletal muscles, circulation and respiration will be examined from the viewpoint of homeothermy. These functions underlie the thermoregulatory responses that fit well within the temporal dimensions of the ultradian sleep cycle of NREM and REM sleep.

Body Temperature

Body temperature is a physical signal of both general physicochemical and specific physiological significance. In other words, body temperature influences directly the cellular life (thermophysical and thermochemical effects) and indirectly the somatic and autonomic activity of the whole organism by excitation of specific thermoreceptors. As a result of the latter influence, thermoregulatory mechanisms maintain a substantial homeothermy of the body core in mammals.

In homeothermic conditions, temperature, as a physical signal, stabilises the physicochemical processes in the body tissues notwithstanding the changes in ambient temperature. The fact that thermoregulatory responses are present or absent depending on the sleep state stresses the operative difference between the general and continuous non-specific action of the physical signal and its sleep state-dependent specific action as a physiological parameter that modulates feedback neural activity for thermoregulation. In the latter case, the peripheral and central thermore-ceptors of the organism are influenced differently by temperature as a consequence of its thermal compartmentalisation in the shell and the core of the body.

The temperatures of the body core (central nervous system and viscera) and the body periphery differ, central temperatures being normally higher and more stable than peripheral temperatures. The information derived from the regional values of temperature is eventually integrated by the control mechanisms that are located in the preoptic–hypothalamic area, which then elicits the somatic and autonomic responses underlying the defence of the homeothermy of the body core.

Homeothermy

There are circadian oscillations of body core temperature in mammals that are relatively small with respect to those of the ambient temperature as a result of the controlled balance between heat production and heat loss. A change in temperature (ΔT) may be quantitatively expressed as the ratio between the change in heat content (ΔQ) and the mass (m) of the tissue multiplied by the specific heat (c) of the tissue ($\Delta T = \Delta Q/mc$). There is a neutral zone of ambient temperature. This zone is defined, on the basis of physiological criteria, as follows: "*The range of ambient temperature at which temperature regulation is achieved only by control of sensible heat loss, i.e., without regulatory changes in metabolic heat production or evaporative heat loss*" (I.U.P.S., 1987, p. 584).

The heat produced by cellular metabolism is transferred to the blood and carried to the systemic heat exchangers of the body (upper airways mucosa, pinna of the ear, tail and glabrous skin). In these regions the controlled vaso-motion adjusts heat dissipation to the environment to maintain the homeothermy of the body core. In theory, core temperature is constant when the heat content of the body is unchanged as the result of a perfect balance between heat production and heat loss to the environment. In reality, perfect homeothermy does not exist. In general, a tachymetabolic (warm-blooded) organism is considered homeothermic when the circadian variation in core temperature "*is maintained within arbitrarily defined limits ($\pm 2°C$) despite much wider variations in ambient temperature*" (I.U.P.S., 1987, p. 574).

This regulatory system involves a set-range of normal core temperatures that defines the boundaries beyond which error signals activate auxiliary thermoregulatory responses in addition to vasomotion.

The afferent discharges from superficial and deep thermoreceptors of the body act as inputs to control the activity of the central thermostat in the preoptic-hypothalamic area and of subordinate brain stem and spinal mechanisms (see Satinoff, 1978). The central thermoregulatory structures are also equipped with thermoresponsive neurons, reacting selectively to central cold and warm thermal stimuli, which are direct feedback inputs to them. The response gain of this feedback regulation shows that small preoptic-hypothalamic temperature deviations from the normal set-range activate thermoregulatory responses (von Euler, 1964).

Physiological Effectors of Thermoregulation

Before approaching the thermoregulatory peculiarities of sleep, it will be helpful to consider briefly the effector mechanisms of thermoregulation in mammalian species. The thermoregulatory responses to external (environment), and internal (body) positive (warm) and negative (cold) thermal loads are either behavioural or autonomic. The rationale for this distinction (I.U.P.S., 1987, p. 581) is explained below.

Behavioural thermoregulation (the term "behavioural" refers to somato-motor and postural activities) influences passive heat loss by means of changes in posture (e.g., curling or sprawling) and/or location (to increase or decrease exposure to sun, wind, humidity, etc.) of the body with respect to the thermal environment.

Autonomic thermoregulation (the term "autonomic" is used in its general sense and does not imply that all responses are controlled by the autonomic nervous system) actively influences both heat production (shivering, non-shivering thermogenesis) and heat loss (vasomotion of heat exchangers, piloerection, thermal tachypnea and sweating).

The behavioural responses are aimed at establishing appropriate ambient conditions affecting the heat exchange of the body with its environment; and the autonomic responses, at affecting directly heat production and heat loss in order to restore the balance between the two variables underlying body core homeothermy.

The ultradian sleep cycle in mammalian species is characterised by specific short-term changes in behavioural and autonomic thermoregulation that have nothing in common with the long-term changes in thermoregulatory responses resulting from the acclimatisation to low or high ambient temperatures.

Behavioural Thermoregulation in Sleep

In wakefulness, the activity of skeletal muscles underlies the basic behaviours of nutrition, behavioural and autonomic (shivering) thermoregulation, reproduction, active (attack) and passive (flight, hiding) defence against all kinds of ambient dangers in order to secure the survival of the organism and the species. Of these behaviours, only passive defence (hiding) and behavioural thermoregulation directly promote sleep onset, and both depend on the activity of skeletal muscles.

In general, mammals display an appetitive pre-sleep behaviour (Parmeggiani, 1968), that is in part species specific and in part influenced by the actual temperature signal at sleep onset. Such defensive behaviour reduces the demand for autonomic temperature regulation during sleep.

There is no reason to enumerate in detail the many preliminary measures devised by animals of different species but a few examples are presented below. Whatever the natural defence against thermal loads may be, it is maintained or varied across NREM sleep in response to ambient temperature, thus providing the sleeping organism with the most favourable thermal condition at low energetic cost.

Both motor and postural patterns characterise the transition from wakefulness to NREM sleep. The motor activity is aimed at finding a safe and thermally comfortable ecological niche to assume the natural sleep posture. The postural attitude is both reactive to the actual ambient temperature and predictive to protect the regulated decrease in body temperature during NREM sleep.

In general, heat loss is regulated according to ambient temperature by decreasing or increasing the surface of the body that is exposed to the surrounding air or the ground (Parmeggiani and Rabini, 1970). In particular, curling up and sprawling influence in opposite ways the abdominal thermal stimulation which modulates, particularly in furry species, the sympathetic vasoconstrictor outflow to the heat exchangers of the body (skin, pinna of the ear, upper airway mucosa and tail) (Azzaroni and Parmeggiani, 1995a,b). Also, inspired air is thermally conditioned by placing the nose either close to or away from the body surface depending on the posture chosen by the animal at low or high ambient temperatures, respectively. The control of inspired air temperature also influences the temperature of the venous blood flowing from the upper airway mucosa to the heart. In some species, such blood contributes to the regulation of the temperature of the brain before returning to the heart, thanks to counter-current or conductive mechanisms of heat exchange with the carotid blood (Hayward and Baker, 1969), which will be described in detail in Chapter 7. Thus, the specific body postures, reduce the energetic cost of homeo-thermy in sleep and provide a thermal condition that is propitious to sleep even when the ambient temperature is outside the ambient thermoneutral zone of the species (see Altman and Dittmer, 1966).

The posture of thermal defence assumed at sleep onset is maintained or modified throughout NREM sleep depending on the persistence or change of the thermal load. In addition, efficient reactive thermoregulation involving skeletal muscles is shown by shivering and thermal tachypnea during NREM sleep. Only under the influence of heavy thermal loads may NREM sleep be interrupted by arousal.

Postural atonia and myoclonic twitches reveal a remarkable change in the neural control of skeletal muscle activity in REM sleep (Jouvet, 1962). Such somatic features are in sharp contrast with the actively maintained quiet postural pattern of NREM sleep. Moreover, the changes in the motor innervation of skeletal muscles occur independently of the ambient tem-perature in REM sleep. The loss of the neural control of the body posture produces small postural changes due to the unchallenged influence of grav-ity on the lying body. Muscle atonia and muscle twitches are due to the tonic inhibition and irregular excitation of the motor neurons innervating the skeletal muscles in REM sleep (see Chase and Morales, 2005).

In conclusion, across the ultradian sleep cycle there is not only a NREM sleep-related suspension of motor activity associated with the maintenance of the thermoregulatory posture, but also a REM sleep-related condition of postural muscle atonia associated with irregular bursts of phasic motor innervation. The phenomena of REM sleep are not only inconsistent with thermoregulation, but also puzzling in terms of general physiological significance.

Autonomic Thermoregulation in Sleep

Pre-sleep behaviour promotes the occurrence of NREM sleep. The intrinsic decrease in metabolic and sympathetic activity of NREM sleep leads to a decrease in heat production (Brebbia and Altshuler, 1965; Haskell et al., 1981; Palca et al., 1986; Webb and Hiestand, 1975) and an increase in heat loss (Azzaroni and Parmeggiani, 1995b). The eventual result is the regulated decrease in core temperature that is typical of this state of sleep. The intensity of tonic vasoconstriction of heat exchangers in quiet wakefulness is decreased during NREM sleep as a sleep-dependent event (Azzaroni and Parmeggiani, 1995b). An increase in heat exchanger temperature and a related increase in brain cooling that lowers preoptic-hypothalamic temperature are the result of such vasodilatation (Azzaroni and Parmeggiani, 1993, 1995a,b; Hayward and Baker, 1969; Parmeggiani et al., 1975). A sharp decline of preoptic-hypothalamic temperature in cats, which is steeper at low ambient temperature than at neutral ambient temperature, has been observed when the head is lowered to assume the sleep posture (Parmeggiani et al., 1975). The head-down posture (decrease in negative hydrostatic load raising the transmural pressure) contributes to the increase in heat exchanger vasodilatation and eventual brain cooling during NREM sleep (Azzaroni and Parmeggiani, 1995a).

In humans, skin vasodilatation in the lower extremities at the onset of NREM sleep (Kräuchi et al., 1997, 1999, 2000; van Someren, 2000) and thermal sweating (Sagot et al., 1987) are phenomena consistent with the down-regulation of body core temperature in this sleep state. The skin vasodilatation reveals a state-dependent change in the central regulation of sympathetic outflow that underlies both a decrease and an increase in vasoconstrictor and vasodilator sympathetic discharge, respectively (Noll et al., 1994). In turn, the resulting increase in skin temperature generates feedforward and feedback effects that further sustain hypothalamic sleep promotion and thermoregulatory skin vasodilatation, respectively. Also artificial moderate warming of the lower extremities may positively influence sleep propensity (Kräuchi et al., 1997, 1999, 2000; van Someren, 2000).

In furry species (e.g., cat, rabbit, rat) the vasodilatation of systemic heat exchangers (pinna of the ear, nasal mucosa) in NREM sleep, as a result of the decrease in sympathetic vasoconstrictor outflow, underlies the decrease in preoptic-hypothalamic temperature (Azzaroni and Parmeggiani, 1993, 1995a,b).

The fact that thermolysis during NREM sleep is controlled by sleep mechanisms was demonstrated by a study in cats (Parmeggiani *et al.*, 1975). The decrease in preoptic-hypothalamic temperature with respect to wakefulness, occurring at the end of the NREM sleep episode of the ultradian sleep cycle, depends quantitatively not only on ambient temperature but also on whether NREM sleep is followed by REM sleep or by arousal. When NREM sleep gives way to REM sleep, the decrease in preoptic-hypothalamic temperature is greater at low (0°C) than at normal (20°C) ambient temperatures. This shows that the functional changes in late NREM sleep underlying REM sleep onset also include a depression in the thermoregulatory control of passive heat loss. In contrast, when NREM sleep is followed by arousal the decrease in hypothalamic temperature is the same at both ambient temperatures showing the maintained efficiency of thermoregulation in late NREM sleep. Therefore, it appears that the onset of REM sleep requires the inactivation of the central thermostat in late NREM sleep. However, only a restricted range of preoptic-hypothalamic temperatures at the end of NREM sleep is compatible with REM sleep onset. This range may be considered a sort of temperature gate for REM sleep, that is constrained in width more at low than at neutral ambient temperature. These results suggest that there is the activation of a process late in NREM sleep that, if overruling the control of the central thermostat, opens the gate to REM sleep onset (NREM–REM sleep switch). Consequently, it appears reasonable that the probability of REM sleep occurrence is the highest at thermal neutrality since the physiological necessity of heat loss during NREM sleep easily prevails, lacking an antagonistic interaction between sleep processes and ambient thermal influences.

Autonomic temperature regulation (vasomotion, piloerection, shivering, thermal tachypnea, sweating) persists during NREM sleep in response to thermal loads without eliciting awakening from sleep. However, the probability of REM sleep occurrence is decreased unless a consistent REM sleep pressure has been accumulated as a result of previous REM sleep suppression in order to maintain the thermoregulatory responses to ambient thermal loads (Parmeggiani and Rabini, 1970; Parmeggiani *et al.*, 1969, 1980). In the long run, however, improving acclimatisation to ambient temperature may restore REM sleep occurrence.

In conclusion, the interaction between REM sleep and thermoregulation features a clear-cut functional antagonism (see Parmeggiani, 1980b). The behavioural and autonomic thermoregulatory responses elicited by ambient thermal loads during NREM sleep are absent during REM sleep.

As already mentioned, posture clearly varies in relation to ambient temperature during NREM sleep, whereas the drop in postural muscle tone during REM sleep is unrelated to ambient temperature (Parmeggiani and Rabini, 1970). As shown by the following experimental results, autonomic thermoregulation is also suspended during REM sleep. Thermal tachypnea in the cat (Parmeggiani and Rabini, 1967) and heat exchanger vasodilation in the cat (Parmeggiani *et al.*, 1977), rabbit (Franzini *et al.*, 1982) and rat (Alföldi *et al.*, 1990) disappear notwithstanding a positive thermal load. Sweating in humans is at first suppressed (Dewasmes *et al.*, 1997) and then depressed (Amoros *et al.*, 1986; Dewasmes *et al.*, 1997; Henane *et al.*, 1977; Sagot *et al.*, 1987; Shapiro *et al.*, 1974) during the episode of REM sleep. Shivering in the cat (Parmeggiani and Rabini, 1967) and armadillo (Affanni *et al.*, 1972; Prudom and Klemm, 1973; van Twyver and Allison, 1974), heat exchanger vasoconstriction in the cat (Parmeggiani *et al.*, 1977), rabbit (Franzini *et al.*, 1982) and rat (Alföldi *et al.*, 1990) and piloerection in the cat (Hendricks, 1982; Hendricks *et al.*, 1977) are suppressed during the REM sleep episode in the presence of a negative thermal load. In addition, the warming function of interscapular brown adipose tissue (BAT) is altered in rats during REM sleep under a negative thermal load (Calasso *et al.*, 1993). This appears to be a result of the sharp decrease in BAT's temperature observed only during REM sleep. The reason is that the cold-defence function of BAT is primarily dependent on a higher temperature than that of the tissues to be thermoregulated.

Concerning the suppression of shivering during REM sleep, a crucial experiment has shown that this occurs also in cats with pontine lesions producing REM sleep without muscle atonia (Hendricks, 1982; Hendricks *et al.*, 1977; see Morrison, 2005). This experiment falsified the objection that the disappearance of shivering in normal conditions is simply a result of the pontine inhibition of spinal motoneurons producing muscle atonia in REM sleep and not a pure expression of the inhibition of thermoregulation at high integrative levels. On this basis, the conclusion is warranted that the suppression of shivering in the intact animal during REM sleep involves also a change in the activity of the proposed hypothalamic neuronal network for thermoregulatory shivering (Kanosue *et al.*, 1994b). The experiment of REM sleep without atonia has other important implications in addition to thermoregulation, which will be considered in Chapter 8.

The vasomotion observed during REM sleep is inconsistent with the control of homeothermy. In particular, an alteration of the autonomic regulation affects particularly the vessels of the systemic heat exchangers (pinna of the ear, nasal mucosa) in furry species (cats, rabbits, rats). As already mentioned, on the transition from NREM sleep to REM sleep, the systemic heat exchangers of such species show that thermoregulatory vasoconstriction is replaced by vasodilatation at low ambient temperature and thermoregulatory vasodilatation by vasoconstriction at high ambient temperature (Parmeggiani *et al.*, 1977; Franzini *et al.*, 1982). During REM sleep, only forehead skin vasodilatation in naked human adults exposed to 21°C ambient temperature is inconsistent with thermoregulation (Palca *et al.*, 1986). However, the study of vasomotion during sleep in naked humans may be insufficiently extensive with regard to the range of negative thermal loads explored, particularly in comparison with the bearable positive thermal loads inducing sweating.

The following experimental results show that the responsiveness of the preoptic-hypothalamic thermostat to direct thermal stimuli is dependent on the state of sleep. The thermoregulatory responses elicited by positive and negative thermal loads applied directly to the thermoreceptive preoptic-anterior hypothalamic area are abolished during REM sleep. In the cat, warming elicits tachypnea (Fig. 7) (Parmeggiani *et al.*, 1973, 1976) and heat exchanger vasodilatation (Fig. 8) (Parmeggiani *et al.*, 1977) during NREM sleep but has no effect during REM sleep. It is interesting to note that arousal from REM sleep immediately reactivates tachypnea (Fig. 9). In the kangaroo, rat (Glotzbach and Heller, 1976) and marmot (Florant *et al.*, 1978), hypothalamic cooling with water-perfused thermodes increases oxygen consumption and metabolic heat production during NREM sleep, whereas it is ineffective during REM sleep.

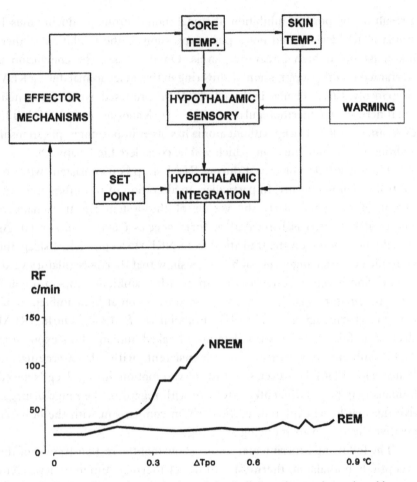

Fig. 7. Influence of preoptic-anterior hypothalamic diathermic warming on breathing rate during sleep (cat). The slope of breathing rate during NREM sleep shows a steep increase beyond the response threshold (about 0.2°C), whereas there is no response during REM sleep. NREM, NREM sleep; REM, REM sleep; RF, respiratory frequency; Tpo, preoptic temperature. (Modified from Parmeggiani *et al.*, 1976.)

The previous data suggest the existence of an effective antagonism between REM sleep processes and thermoregulation in the control of somatic and autonomic effector mechanisms also at the high integrative levels of the nervous system. Such interaction is evidenced by preoptic-anterior hypothalamic thermoresponsive neurons showing changes in their

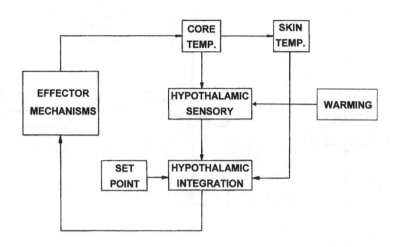

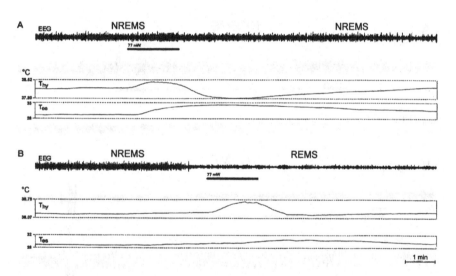

Fig. 8. Influence of preoptic-anterior hypothalamic diathermic warming on the temperature of the pinna of the ear during sleep at ambient thermal neutrality (cat). A: warming
increases hypothalamic temperature at first and subsequently the temperature of the pinna
of the ear in NREMS. During the latter increase, there is a fall of hypothalamic temperature
below the control level as a result of blood cooling due to the heat exchanger vasodilatation.
B: warming does not affect the late slight spontaneous increment of ear pinna temperature
occurring normally at this ambient temperature in REMS. EEG, electroencephalogram;
mW, milliwatt; NREMS, NREM sleep; REMS, REM sleep; Thy, hypothalamic
temperature; Tes, ear skin temperature. (Modified from Parmeggiani *et al.*, 1977.)

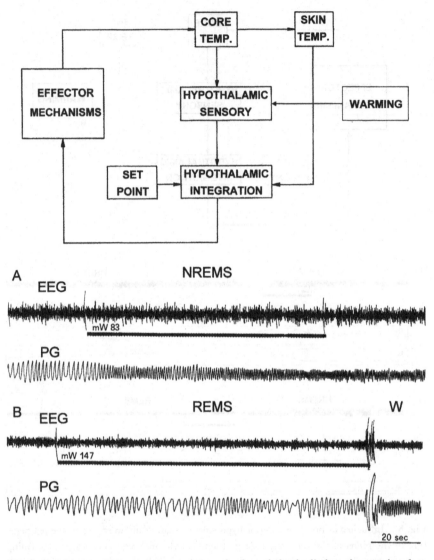

Fig. 9. Respiratory responses to preoptic-anterior hypothalamic diathermic warming during sleep (cat). A: warming elicits tachypnea which persists also after the end of warming in NREMS. B: warming is ineffective during REMS notwithstanding the increased intensity. Tachypnea starts immediately with the arousal of the animal. EEG, electroencephalogram; mW, milliwatt; NREMS, NREM sleep; PG, pneumogram; REMS, REM sleep; W, wakefulness. (Modified from Parmeggiani *et al.*, 1973.)

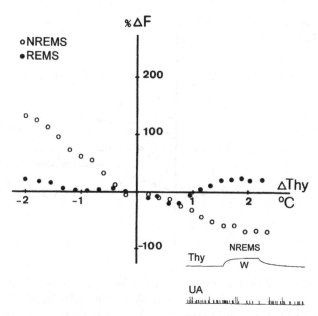

Fig. 10. Firing rate of a cold-responsive neuron as a function of changes (water perfused thermode) in preoptic-anterior hypothalamic temperature in NREM sleep (open circles) and REM sleep (filled circles) (cat). The insert shows the inhibition of firing (ordinate: 0–3 spikes/s) elicited by warming (W) during NREMS. ΔF, relative frequency change of firing with respect to base line; ΔThy, hypothalamic temperature change (°C); UA, unit activity. (Modified from Parmeggiani *et al.*, 1987.)

thermal characteristics across the ultradian sleep cycle (Alam *et al.*, 1995a,b, 1997, 2002; Glotzbach and Heller, 1984; McGinty *et al.*, 2001, 2005; Parmeggiani *et al.*, 1983, 1986, 1987). In particular, the lower responsiveness of a cold-responsive neuron (Fig. 10) with respect to a warm-responsive neuron (Fig. 11) to direct thermal stimulation in NREM sleep appears consistent with the down-regulation of body and brain temperatures in this state of sleep. In REM sleep, both neurons are not responsive to the specific thermal stimulus.

REM sleep mechanisms override the specific activity of the preoptic-hypothalamic thermoreceptive network underlying thermoregulation. In the cat, the body temperature increased and decreased in a warm and cold environment, respectively (Parmeggiani *et al.*, 1971). In other words, the

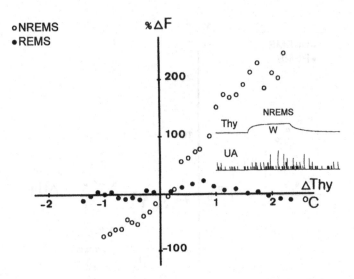

Fig. 11. Firing rate of a warm-responsive neuron as a function of changes (water perfused thermode) in preoptic-anterior hypothalamic temperature in NREM sleep (open circles) and REM sleep (filled circles) (cat). The insert shows the increase of firing (ordinate: 0–10 spikes/s) elicited by warming (W) during NREMS. ΔF, relative frequency change of firing with respect to base line; ΔThy, hypothalamic temperature change (°C); UA, unit activity. (Modified from Parmeggiani *et al.*, 1987.)

changes in body temperature during REM sleep are positively correlated with ambient temperature, as expected in poikilothermic species (Fig. 12).

In the presented case, the rate of change of body temperature during REM sleep in the cold environment (−15°C) was 0.0017°C/min·°C(T_B−T_A) (T_A, ambient temperature; T_B, body temperature) in a normal cat during REM sleep (Parmeggiani *et al.*, 1971). In a poikilothermic pontine preparation the rate was 0.0027°C/min·°C(T_B−T_A) (calculated from data of Bard *et al.*, 1970). This change in REM sleep amounts to about 62.96% of the pontine preparation. There are other compelling proofs of a positive correlation between body core temperature and ambient temperature during REM sleep according to the thermal inertia of the species. In the pocket mouse, above and below the ambient thermal neutrality of this species, the hypothalamic temperature increased and decreased, respectively, during REM

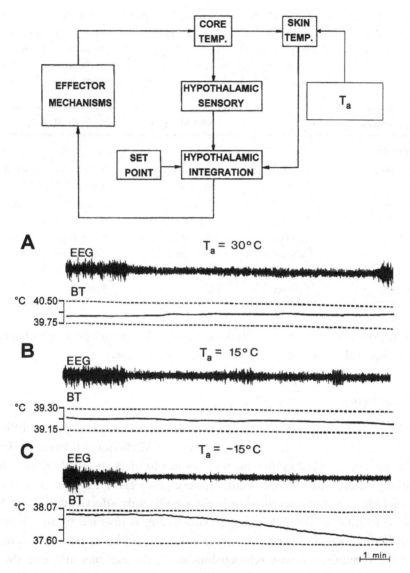

Fig. 12. Changes in body temperature during REM sleep at different environmental temperatures (cat). Body temperature (inguinal subcutaneous temperature) slightly increases at moderately high ambient temperature (A, 30°C), slightly decreases at moderately low ambient temperature (B, 15°C), remarkably decreases at very low ambient temperature (C, −15°C). BT, body temperature; EEG, electroencephalogram; Ta, ambient temperature. (Modified from Parmeggiani *et al.*, 1971.)

Table 3. Thermoregulation during the ultradian wake–sleep cycle. Behavioural and autonomic thermoregulation are present during wakefulness and NREM sleep and absent during REM sleep in furry species. During REM sleep in humans, sweating is at first abolished and then depressed. Specific: thermoregulatory responses; Non-specific: alarm responses; Wake, wakefulness; NREM sleep, non-rapid-eye-movement sleep; REM sleep, rapid-eye-movement sleep.

Responses	Wake	NREM sleep	REM sleep
Specific			
Behavioural	Locomotion	No locomotion	No locomotion, twitches
	Posture	Tonic posture	Atonic posture
Autonomic	Vasomotion	Vasomotion	Inconsistent vasomotion
	Piloerection	Piloerection	No piloerection
	Shivering	Shivering	No shivering
	Tachypnea	Tachypnea	No tachypnea
	Sweating	Sweating	Sweating (0,–)
Non-specific	Vigilance	Arousal	Arousal

sleep (Walker *et al.*, 1983). Table 3 summarises the thermoregulatory characteristics of the states of the ultradian wake–sleep cycle.

Conclusion

The experimental results have shown that there are species specific differences of the sleep states from the viewpoint of thermoregulation. A few differences observed in humans with respect to furry species deserve to be briefly considered in more detail. However, they are not crucial enough to conclude that thermoregulation is not significantly affected during REM sleep in human adults. Caution in concluding is justified by the several methodological constraints impeding in human adults an exhaustive study of the stimulus–response relationships of all the variables affecting thermoregulation during sleep. From the physiological viewpoint, moreover, there is a remarkable difference between human adults and small furry mammals concerning thermal inertia and insulation, specific heat exchanger surface and skin area as source of sensory inputs. On the other hand, suppression and depression of sweating and forehead skin vasodilatation during REM sleep under positive and negative thermal loads, respectively, are changes suggesting at least a depression in the excitatory drive of the preoptic-hypothalamic thermostat on the subordinate mechanisms: a drive necessarily underlying normal thermoregulatory responses.

From a functional viewpoint, a reasonable inference is that a highly integrated autonomic thermoregulation is necessary in furry mammals characterised by small specific heat exchanger surfaces and small thermal inertia. In contrast, the lack of fur insulation and a large thermal inertia would be consistent with a less centralised thermoregulatory control that is also based on reflex mechanisms at lower levels of the neuraxis (see Satinoff, 1978) for autonomous regional regulation of heat loss (vasomotion and sweating) and production (shivering). This view may be consistent with the fact that thermal tachypnea, as a normal thermoregulatory response, is not present in human adults. The lack of thermal tachypnea is not really surprising from the teleological viewpoint. In a species devoid of fur, sweating is a most effective cause of heat loss that does not require the activation of respiratory muscles and does not conflict with another function of breathing (phonation) having also high priority in humans.

In conclusion, it is reasonable to accept that an alteration of the preoptic-hypothalamic regulation of homeothermy affects in different ways all the studied mammals during REM sleep. In other words, this event is less evident and dramatic in humans than in other mammalian species probably as a result of a different hierarchical organisation of the thermoregulatory mechanisms. Considering the human newborn, a reliable comparison with the human adult is not possible since the evolution of sleep with its states of NREM sleep and REM sleep has not yet occurred. There is no consensus whether quiet sleep and active sleep observed in the newborn correspond to NREM sleep and REM sleep, respectively. In addition, many thermoregulatory mechanisms are still immature, although a thermoregulatory defence particularly against negative thermal loads is state specific. The increase in duration of active sleep is associated with enhanced heat production by the brown adipose tissue and also increased muscular activity (see Libert and Bach, 2005).

To sum up, the experimental results presented in this chapter show the existence in mammals of a radical dichotomy in the control of body temperature between NREM sleep and REM sleep. The first is a homeothermic state as a result of behavioural and autonomic thermoregulation, whereas the second is characterised by the suspension of both behavioural and autonomic thermoregulation. For this reason, REM sleep cannot be considered merely a poikilothermic (ectothermic) state, since poikilothermic species are those in which body temperature depends on behavioural thermoregulation. Since this is not the case with REM sleep lacking both behavioural and autonomic thermoregulation, this state is better characterised by the qualification "*poikilostatic*" that includes also its variable respiratory and circulatory phenomenology. Such qualification points out the state-dependent persistence (static) of the functional modality (*poikilo* = disintegrated physiological functions) of systemic unstable physiological regulation.

Chapter 6

Influence of Temperature on Sleep

In the previous chapter, body temperature was considered a physical variable having the role of a physiological parameter from the viewpoint of the control of body homeothermy during sleep. In this section, ambient temperature is considered as a physical variable having the role of an important ambient cue for sleep expression. This will complete the picture of the exceedingly tight and complex internal and external interaction between the variable temperature and the neural mechanisms underlying sleep. In short, as sleep affects thermoregulation, so thermoregulation affects sleep.

Concerning the role of temperature as an ambient cue for sleep expression, the experimental data show that ambient thermal loads antagonise and postpone particularly the onset of REM sleep. NREM sleep is obviously less affected by ambient temperature unless the thermal load is heavy. It is understandable, therefore, why a thermoneutral environment, requiring no energetically expensive responses for thermoregulation, promotes the occurrence of a complete ultradian sleep cycle.

Influence of Ambient Temperature on the Ultradian Wake–Sleep Cycle

The structure of the ultradian wake–sleep cycle at ambient temperatures within the thermoneutral zone is conventionally considered the normal reference. The thermoneutral zone, which varies among the different species (see Altman and Dittmer, 1966), is the range of ambient temperatures within which the metabolic expense for thermoregulation decreases to a minimum at rest. Within this range, temperature regulation is implemented by physical mechanisms (conductive, convective, radiant heat loss) and by vasomotion in the heat exchangers. Stated otherwise, the thermoneutral zone is "*The range of ambient temperature at which tempera-ture regulation is achieved only by control of sensible heat loss, i.e., without regulatory changes in metabolic heat production or evaporative heat loss*" (I.U.P.S., 1987, p. 584). The amount of thermal load does not only depend on ambient temperature: other factors, such as humidity, body size, ther-mal insulation, age, sexual cycle, feeding, season, etc. as well as differences in regional body sensitivity to temperature, consistently influence individ-ual thermoregulatory responses. Acclimatisation to ambient temperatures beyond the limits of the thermoneutral zone induces shifts and/or modifi-cations of the ambient temperature range well tolerated by various species in terms of normal structure and duration of the ultradian wake–sleep cycle (Parmeggiani and Rabini, 1970; Parmeggiani et al., 1969). The set of interacting variables, therefore, is complex from both behavioural and physiological viewpoints. Figure 13 shows the cumulative duration of wakefulness (and reciprocally of sleep) in a cat exposed in the winter to different air temperatures in a thermoregulated box during a diurnal period of 12 h of artificial light. In this season the minimum duration of wakefulness

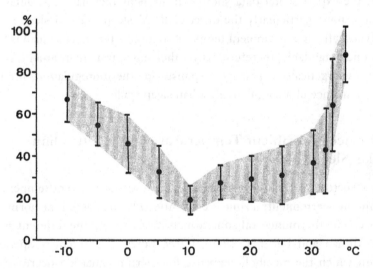

Fig. 13.   Relative duration (mean and SD) of wakefulness in a cat, exposed to different air temperatures in a thermoregulated box, during the diurnal period (12 h of artificial light) in winter. In the same cat, the minimal amount of wakefulness corresponded to an air temperature of 25°C in summer. (Modified from Parmeggiani, 2005b.)

was observed at 10°C, whereas it was found at 25°C air temperature in the summer. This shows the effects of acclimatisation on the thermal insulation of the body. In other words, the increase or the decrease of the thermal protection exerted by the fur influences also the thermoneutral range of sleep (Parmeggiani, 2005b).

Maximal sleep duration occurs within the ambient thermoneutrality range (Obal *et al.*, 1983; Parmeggiani and Rabini, 1970; Sakaguchi *et al.*, 1979; Schmidek *et al.*, 1972; Sichieri and Schmidek, 1984; Valatx *et al.*, 1973) and peaks at its upper limit (Szymusiak and Satinoff, 1981). Waking time increases above and below this range but the rate of increase is larger above than below it.

The increase in waking time without the thermoneutral range is directly related to the rate of increase in energy expenditure for temperature regulation (Hensel *et al.*, 1973, p. 533). On the other hand, the correlation between brain weight and sleep cycle length is positive (see Zepelin, 2000), when no exogenous factors (e.g., nutritional habit, ecological niche, predator–prey relationship) prevail over thermoregulation by affecting the survival conditions of the species. This suggests that the structure of the ultradian sleep cycle, particularly with regard to NREM sleep and REM sleep episode duration, also depends on the thermal inertia of the brain and secondarily of the body (see Zepelin, 2000). This inertia influences the time course of changes in the internal temperature signal affecting sleep processes.

The deviations of ambient temperature from thermoneutrality, which increase the waking time, also modify the structure of sleep (Haskell *et al.*, 1981; Parmeggiani and Rabini, 1970; Parmeggiani *et al.*, 1969; Sakaguchi *et al.*, 1979; Schmidek *et al.*, 1972; Sewitch *et al.*, 1986; Sichieri and Schmidek, 1984; Szymusiak and Satinoff, 1981). In particular, NREM sleep and/or REM sleep may be selectively affected depending on the quality and intensity of the thermal load. Outside the thermoneutrality range, REM sleep in particular is progressively depressed and eventually suppressed (Cerri *et al.*, 2005; Haskell *et al.*, 1981; Parmeggiani and Rabini, 1970; Parmeggiani *et al.*, 1969, 1974; Sakaguchi *et al.*, 1979; Szymusiak and Satinoff, 1981). However, the accumulation of an increasing REM sleep debt produces sufficient REM sleep pressure to overwhelm periodically the thermoregulatory drive of the preoptic-hypothalamic thermostat

(Parmeggiani, 1987; Parmeggiani and Rabini, 1970; Parmeggiani *et al.*, 1969, 1974, 1980). In this case, the brain stem effector mechanisms of REM sleep functionally escape from the normal preoptic-hypothalamic control, and thermoregulatory responses are temporarily suppressed. Nevertheless, the organism is not endangered in REM sleep since the loss of the specific thermoregulatory effects of thermal stimuli is not associated with a loss of their non-specific arousing influence, which re-establishes full somatic and autonomic thermoregulatory functions (see Table 3 in Chapter 5).

Two types of REM sleep episodes have been identified in rats. The "single episode" is preceded and followed by a long interval without REM sleep of more than 3 minutes, and the "cluster," which occurs as a sequence of REM sleep episodes (sequential episodes) separated by very short intervals of less than or equal to 3 minutes (Amici *et al.*, 1994). The cluster of sequential REM sleep episodes has an average duration almost double than that of a single episode. In small animals with a high surface to volume ratio there is a tendency to modulate the circadian amount of REM sleep more in terms of episode frequency than duration under the influence of different ambient temperatures (Amici *et al.*, 1994, 1998; Roussel *et al.*, 1980; Sakaguchi *et al.*, 1979; Sichieri and Schmidek, 1984; Zamboni *et al.*, 2001).

The single episode of REM sleep is less depressed by negative thermal loads than the sequential episodes (Zamboni *et al.*, 1997). This shows that the iterative switch mechanism of the REM cluster is more depressed by thermal loads than that of the switch of single episodes (see Amici *et al.*, 2005). On this basis, the functional significance of the arousal episodes intermingled in the REM sleep cluster may not concern primarily the control of homeothermy under thermal loads. The possibility deserves consideration that predated species of small size utilise the short arousal between sequential REM sleep episodes to control the environment at ambient thermal neutrality when the maximum of REM sleep is attained either in normal or recovery conditions after deprivation. Concerning the control of the environment, a thermal challenge anyhow increases the duration of wakefulness, and consequently the control of the environment, to protect homeothermy. In such condition, however, the increasing REM sleep debt promotes only single episodes of this state that reduce periodically the pressure of such debt. Only after return to the neutral range of ambient temperature the recovery of REM sleep is characterised by a predominant number of clusters with respect to that of single episodes.

In conclusion, complex interactions between several important exogenous and endogenous influences (temperature, ecological niche, predator–prey relationship, feeding and sexual drives) and REM sleep expression underlie the changes in the structure of the ultradian wake–sleep cycle and particularly the modality of REM sleep occurrence in different species.

Experimentally induced changes in the preoptic-anterior hypothalamic temperature also affect the ultradian wake–sleep cycle. Cooling increases waking time (Sakaguchi *et al.*, 1979), and moderate warming promotes both NREM and REM sleep (von Euler and Söderberg, 1957; Parmeggiani *et al.*, 1974, 1980; Roberts and Robinson, 1969; Roberts *et al.*, 1969; Sakaguchi *et al.*, 1979). Such effects probably depend on the specific thermoregulatory features of sleep behaviour. The thermoregulatory activity elicited by either a cold ambient or preoptic-anterior hypothalamic cooling is practically the opposite of the thermolytic adjustments, such as heat exchanger vasodilatation associated with decrease in metabolic heat production, that are induced by NREM sleep processes. In contrast, a moderately warm ambient or preoptic-anterior hypothalamic warming strengthens sleep promotion. Such conditions induce somatic effects, such as muscle hypotonia and postural heat loss, and autonomic effects, such as heat exchanger vasodilatation and sweating, that are synergistic with the influence of NREM sleep executive control on the same effector mechanisms. On the other hand, a balance between opposing ambient and preoptic-anterior hypothalamic thermal loads influencing peripheral and central thermoreceptors, respectively, may be experimentally achieved so as to promote sleep. In particular, warming of the preoptic-anterior hypothalamic region in a cold environment hastens REM sleep onset and increases its duration (Parmeggiani *et al.*, 1974, 1980; Sakaguchi *et al.*, 1979). The antagonistic interaction between warm- and cold-stimuli, applied concomitantly at peripheral and central levels, is also evident in the activity of thermoresponsive neurons during sleep (Cevolani and Parmeggiani, 1995).

The relationship between sleep processes and thermoregulation at high integration levels is intimate. For example, the changes in activity of preoptic-anterior hypothalamic warm-responsive neurons across quiet wakefulness, NREM and REM sleep are also consistent with a direct involvement of such neurons in sleep regulation (Alam et al., 1995a,b, 1997, 2002; McGinty et al., 2001; Szymusiak et al., 2001). In particular, there are thermoresponsive neurons, also activated by peripheral thermoreceptors, in the median preoptic nucleus and ventrolateral preoptic area which show increasing activity at sleep onset or in response to increase in core and/or skin temperatures. These neurons release inhibitory neurotransmitters (GABA, galanin) inhibiting neurons in the perifornical lateral and posterior hypothalamus (orexinergic/hypocretinergic), dorsal raphe nucleus (serotonergic), locus coeruleus (noradrenergic) and brain stem and basal forebrain systems (cholinergic) underlying arousal mechanisms. Conversely, cold sensitive neurons underlie the activation of the system of neurons underlying the arousal mechanisms opposing the onset of sleep. In conclusion the preoptic-anterior hypothalamic neurons may represent a neurophysiological substrate for the sleep-promoting influence of ambient or preoptic-hypothalamic moderate warming (see McGinty et al., 2005).

The functional interaction between thermoregulation and sleep, appears also in the c-Fos expression of the ventrolateral and the median preoptic nucleus during cold exposure inducing sleep deprivation and the following recovery of sleep at neutral ambient temperature in rats (Dentico et al., 2009). During cold exposure, c-Fos expression increased in both nuclei except the T-cluster of the ventrolateral preoptic nucleus. During sleep recovery, c-Fos expression was high in both nuclei and specifically in T-cluster. A still open question, however, is whether c-Fos expression, a marker of neuronal activity, results from either thermoregulatory activation or sleep pressure, or from both factors.

The evidence that thermoregulatory and sleep processes interact agonistically inside and antagonistically outside ambient thermal neutrality points to the importance of the predictive function of the behavioural thermoregulation to sustain normal occurrence of the ultradian sleep cycle. The onset of a pre-sleep behaviour consistent with the ambient thermal load protects at low energy cost the free occurrence of preoptic-anterior hypothalamic temperature changes physiologically bound up with NREM sleep processes. The passive defence of homeothermy during NREM sleep and particularly REM sleep is the more effective the larger the thermal inertia of the body since the specific physiological changes of sleep can occur undisturbed by an imperative demand for autonomic temperature regulation. This demand would entail increased energy expenditure in NREM sleep up to an arousal at the onset of or in REM sleep to overcome the deficit in thermoregulation in this behavioural state. In other words, a successful constraint on energy expenditure for thermoregulation is a requisite for the normal development of the ultradian sleep cycle.

Conclusion

As sleep influences thermoregulation, so thermoregulation influences sleep. The experimental data show that their interaction might bring about the temporary prevalence of either sleep or wakefulness depending on the amount of cumulative sleep deprivation and of the thermal load, respectively. In normal conditions, however, the intermediate situations prevail: NREM sleep and thermoregulation are compatible; and REM sleep and thermoregulation are incompatible. This functional contradiction underlies the variety of outcomes of the interaction of the two processes affecting the structure of the ultradian and circadian sleep cycles.

The study of the interaction between thermoregulatory and sleep processes has revealed a number of systemic physiological phenomena of great consistency which have stood the test of time. However, further important questions are raised by such observations. The deficit in homeostasis (homeostatic debt) occurring during REM sleep is basically different from that of active wakefulness. In the latter case, the debt is real but temporary (e.g., acidosis, hyperthermia during muscle exercise) since it is due to volitional and instinctive drives competing with still operative homeostatic mechanisms. The purpose of the homeostatic debt assumed in active wakefulness is, therefore, teleologically consistent also in terms of homeostasis, since it is aimed at the survival of the organism or the species. In contrast, REM sleep is physiologically inconsistent as a real poikilostatic state. However, this state of sleep is *de facto* physiologically characterised by a homeostatic debt that is almost virtual as a result of the constraints imposed by a short duration that prevents the debt from becoming actual. Therefore, the quality and quantity of the homeostatic debt of REM sleep is not comparable with that of active wakefulness. The condition of poikilostasis of REM sleep in the adult mammal, in spite of its endowed precise homeostatic mechanisms, appears as constitutional and, therefore, not as a result of an accidental or unfortunate deficit in the evolution of homeostatic physiological regulation. It is instead a cogent expression of a basic and still rather mysterious functional need of the nervous system (see Chapter 8) with which it is possible to cope only during a short and quickly reversible suspension of the integrative neural regulation of the physiological functions of the body.

Chapter 7

Compartmentalised Brain Homeostasis in Sleep

The previous chapters present the experimental data concerning the changes during sleep states of the neural regulation of respiration and circulation (Chapters 3, 4), and the interaction between sleep and temperature (Chapters 5, 6). The experimental results demonstrate two different modalities of neural control of these functions: homeostatic in NREM sleep and poikilostatic in REM sleep.

This chapter deals with the influence of sleep-dependent changes in the activity of the systemic physiological operators on the homeostasis of the brain itself. In other words, the issue under scrutiny is how much the neural controller (the brain) is in turn affected by the changes it has imposed on the activity of the basic operators of systemic body homeostasis. The issues of the control of brain temperature and blood flow during sleep will be considered only regarding small, furry species (cat, rabbit and rat) because these species have been experimentally studied more than others in this respect.

There is a substantial thermal equilibrium of brain temperature across sleep states since it decreases in NREM sleep and increases in REM sleep by only a few tenths of °C within a wide range of ambient temperatures (Parmeggiani *et al.*, 1975, 1984). It is worth recalling here that an operative central thermostat decreases brain temperature during NREM sleep, whereas the small temperature increase in REM sleep depends on systemic hemodynamic events that are examined in detail below. However, the cerebral blood flow always meets the different metabolic request of the two sleep states.

The mechanisms underlying the compartmentalised control of thermal and circulatory homeostasis of the brain, practically maintained also in REM sleep, are several. In particular, they are: (i) pre-sleep behaviour; (ii) the thermal inertia of body and brain; (iii) the duration of the REM sleep episode; (iv) the interaction between metabolic rate, blood flow and temperature in the neural tissue. Concerning the last mechanism (iv), the brain temperature depends on the interaction between warming by metabolic heat production and cooling by the arterial blood supplied to the brain, while blood flow is directly coupled with brain metabolism (see Franzini, 1992; Maquet, 2000).

Physiological Mechanisms Underlying Brain Cooling

Conductive heat loss from the brain to the environment is essentially irrelevant for brain cooling because of the good thermal insulation. Several layers of different tissues (meninges, cranial bones, scalp or furry skin) protect the brain against conductive heat loss. The heat produced by cellular energy metabolism is mainly transferred to the arterial blood in inverse quantitative relation to its temperature, which is lower than that of the brain in the normal condition (Hayward and Baker, 1969). In other words, the brain's temperature depends on its regulation of body temperature.

There are different vascular mechanisms for cooling the brain in mammals and more than a single mechanism may be operative depending on the species (Fig. 14).

In general, the cool venous blood flowing from the systemic heat exchangers of the body (upper airway mucosa, pinna of the ear, horn, tail and skin, according to the species) to the heart mixes with the warm venous blood returning to the heart from heat-producing body tissues. This systemic mechanism cools the arterial blood, including that flowing to the brain (*systemic brain cooling*). In addition to systemic brain cooling, there are also mechanisms for *selective brain cooling*. The carotid blood supply to the brain is also thermally conditioned in the cat, dog, sheep and goat (Hayward, 1968; Hayward and Baker, 1969) prior to entering into the circle of Willis. Counter-current heat exchange occurs between the arterial blood of the carotid rete and the venous blood of the venous sinuses

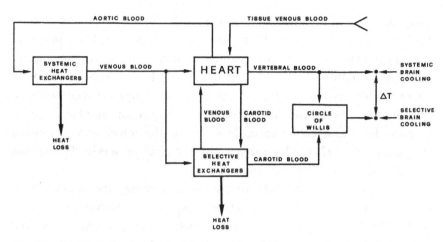

Fig. 14. Diagram showing the mechanisms of systemic and selective brain cooling. Only the routes of blood flow thermally relating systemic and selective heat exchangers with the heart and the encephalon are indicated. The cool venous blood returning to the heart from systemic heat exchangers (pinna of the ear, and nasal mucosa) mixes with warm venous blood returning from body tissues. Vertebral arterial blood is warmer than the carotid arterial blood entering the circle of Willis since the latter is additionally cooled by the selective heat exchangers (e.g., carotid rete-venous plexus). (Modified from Azzaroni and Parmeggiani, 1995a.)

(e.g., *sinus cavernosus*). The carotid rete is a network of fine vessels derived from the external branch of the common carotid artery. The arterial blood flowing to the brain in the carotid rete is surrounded by sinus venous blood cooled in the upper airway mucosa and flowing in an opposite direction toward the heart (Baker and Hayward, 1967a,b; Edvinsson *et al.*, 1993; Hayward and Baker, 1969). The carotid rete is connected to the circle of Willis through a short artery (homologous to the distal part of the internal carotid artery of species lacking the carotid rete, such as the rabbit and rat). As a result of the counter-current heat exchange, the temperature of the carotid blood reaching the circle of Willis is further decreased with respect to that of the aortic arch blood (Baker and Hayward, 1967a,b; Hayward and Baker, 1969). Vertebral artery blood is not thermally conditioned by a counter-current heat-exchange mechanism and enters into the circle of Willis at the temperature of the blood in the aortic arch (Hayward and Baker, 1969). Thus, the difference between the temperatures of vertebral artery blood (systemic cooling only) and carotid artery blood (both systemic and selective cooling) flowing into the circle of Willis depends on the heat loss from the carotid rete. Eventually, the average brain temperature is determined by the relative amounts of carotid and vertebral artery blood contributing to the total blood flow of the brain. Selective brain cooling is also provided by conductive heat exchange between the basal portion of the brain, including the circle of Willis, and the basal venous sinuses that drain cool venous blood from the upper airway mucosa (Caputa et al., 1976). This mechanism is typical of species lacking the carotid rete (e.g., rabbit and rat).

The effect of systemic and selective brain cooling appears in the temperatures of the hindbrain and forebrain, respectively. Pontine temperature is higher than hypothalamic temperature in cats (Azzaroni and Parmeggiani, 1993; Parmeggiani et al., 1998), rabbits (Parmeggiani et al., 1998, 2002) and rats (Calasso and Parmeggiani, 2004; Parmeggiani et al., 1998). Heat loss from systemic heat exchangers, affecting carotid blood temperature through the systemic venous return to the heart (systemic brain cooling), is the most important determinant of brain temperature in primates (Hayward and Baker, 1968, 1969).

The analysis of a physiological parameter, such as brain temperature, and a physiological operator, such as brain blood flow, cannot be carried out independently from each other. The two variables are functionally interrelated and ought to be considered together in order to approach two important mechanisms of compartmentalised brain homeostasis in REM sleep. In the following two sections the analysis focuses first on temperature and then on blood flow.

Defence of Brain Homeothermy in Sleep

Pre-sleep behaviour corresponds exactly to the operational definition of behavioural temperature regulation both for animals and humans (see Chapter 5). This behaviour provides thermoneutral conditions for the sleeping organism also when ambient temperature does not correspond exactly to the ambient thermoneutral zone for the species (see Altman and Dittmer 1966). It has already been pointed out (see Chapters 5 and 6) that such a zone is defined on the basis of physiological criteria, that is, *the range of ambient temperature at which temperature regulation is achieved only by control of sensible heat loss, i.e., without regulatory changes in metabolic heat production or evaporative heat loss* (I.U.P.S., 1987, p. 584). The reason why this thermal condition is so necessary for the free occurrence of "normal" sleep depends on the particular metabolic and autonomic activity during sleep that will be considered next.

Body and brain temperatures decrease during NREM sleep as a result of the decrease in metabolic heat production and the increase in heat loss (see Chapter 5). Concerning heat loss, in quiet wakefulness the vascular heat exchangers are regulated by the vasoconstrictor sympathetic outflow that varies in intensity depending on ambient and/or preoptic-hypothalamic thermal loads. In contrast, during NREM sleep, whatever the actual intensity of tonic vasoconstrictor sympathetic outflow to heat exchangers may be, there is always a decrease in intensity with respect to quiet wakefulness in the cat, a sleep-dependent event in other words (Azzaroni and Parmeggiani, 1995a). The resulting vasodilatation is manifested by an increase in heat exchanger temperature and a related increase in brain cooling that lowers brain temperature during NREM sleep (Azzaroni and Parmeggiani, 1993, 1995b; Hayward and Baker, 1969; Parmeggiani *et al.*, 1975). Also, the head-down posture (decrease in negative hydrostatic load raising the transmural pressure) contributes to increased heat exchanger vasodilatation and the eventual brain cooling during NREM sleep (Azzaroni and Parmeggiani, 1995b; Parmeggiani *et al.*, 1975).

The decrease in metabolic rate and the increase in heat loss are regulated physiological features of NREM sleep (Azzaroni and Parmeggiani, 1995a; Sagot *et al.*, 1987), as result of changes in the preoptic-hypothalamic set point temperature. However, in the case of significant thermal loads, autonomic temperature regulation may also be normally activated during NREM sleep without eliciting immediate awakening from sleep.

The increase in brain temperature in REM sleep is also small (up to a few tenths of a degree Celsius). It is not the expression of thermoregulatory control, however, as is the decrease in brain temperature observed in NREM sleep, but the significant effect of the poikilostatic state of REM sleep. The brain temperature increase in REM sleep is the result of changes in the arterial blood supply to the brain that shall be dealt with in the next section of this chapter.

In conclusion, the decrease in brain temperature in NREM sleep depends on a change in set-point temperature of the thermostat. Therefore, no error load is produced to influence preoptic-hypothalamic thermoresponsive neurons that are still excited by adequate thermal stimulation in NREM sleep (Alam *et al.*, 1995a; Glotzbach and Heller, 1984; Parmeggiani *et al.*, 1983, 1986, 1987). In contrast, the hypothalamic temperature increase in REM sleep cannot be due to active thermoregulation, primarily because the responsiveness of a majority of the preoptic-hypothalamic thermoresponsive neurons is conspicuously depressed during this state of sleep (Alam *et al.*, 1995b; Glotzbach and Heller, 1984; Parmeggiani *et al.*, 1983, 1986, 1987).

The practical question to ask is how the physiological needs for sleep and homeothermy are reconciled. On the basis of the previous considerations, it appears likely that for NREM sleep the operational answer to this question is mainly given by the behavioural temperature regulation displayed at the onset of sleep. Such predictive regulation may be considered also the guardian of REM sleep onset because during NREM sleep it can provide the body with thermal conditions akin to those of ambient thermoneutrality. Therefore, the physiological changes induced by REM sleep processes occur unopposed by the demand for autonomic temperature regulation.

Another factor maintaining the oscillations of hypothalamic temperature within a width of a few tenths of a degree across the ultradian sleep cycle is that the heat generated in the brain by cellular metabolism is transferred to the cooler arterial blood (Azzaroni and Parmeggiani, 1993, 1995b; Hayward and Baker, 1969). In theory, the temperature of the brain is constant when the heat content is unchanged as a result of a perfect balance between heat production and heat loss. In reality, such perfect homeothermy occurs neither in the neural tissue nor in other body tissues. The temperature may be affected by sleep-dependent positive or negative systemic imbalances between heat production and heat loss due to changes in body metabolic rate and in the thermal conductance of heat exchangers. However, such transient imbalances scarcely influence arterial blood temperature since they are efficiently buffered, at no energy cost, by the thermal inertia of the body. Such inertia depends primarily on the high thermal capacity of the mass of body water and the skin's thermal conductance in relation to both the ratio of body surface to body mass and seasonal factors. Among the latter factors, reciprocal changes in the amount of fat and fur with respect to ambient temperature in summer and winter affect heat loss.

The conspicuous role of thermal inertia in the maintenance of the stability of brain temperature is shown by the changes of core temperature during REM sleep in a cat exposed to warm and cold environments. For instance (Parmeggiani *et al.*, 1971), the drop in body core temperature, at $-15°C$ ambient temperature, amounted to $0.4°C$ at the end of a 10 min long REM sleep episode occurring in response to a long term deprivation due to cold exposure. In this case, ambient temperature was about 40°C below the ambient thermal neutrality of the species (Altman and Dittmer, 1966). It is worth noting that the sleep-cycle duration is positively correlated with the weight either of body and brain together or of brain alone, but not of body alone (see Zepelin, 2000). Other exogenous factors (nutritional habits, ecological niche, predator–prey relationship) affecting the survival of the species may disrupt this correlation. However, it is reasonable to consider at least the following hypothesis. This correlation may reveal a phylogenetic pressure. There is a biological advantage of fitting the duration of the ultradian sleep cycle, and particularly that of REM sleep episodes, to the thermal inertia of the organism and particularly of the brain to keep down the energy expenditure for temperature regulation to promote sleep.

To sum up, the homeothermy of the brain is protected, by general active and passive defense mechanisms, such as pre-sleep behaviour and thermal inertia of brain and body that operate at a low energy cost to promote normal sleep occurrence. These mechanisms are capable of maintaining preoptic-hypothalamic temperature within the neutral zone of the central thermostat, that is, with only a subliminal error load with respect to set point temperature notwithstanding the considerable range of thermal loads in natural environments. The most important active defence of homeothermy in NREM sleep is predictive, as it is set before sleep by behavioural temperature regulation. This behaviour provides thermal conditions counteracting the static influence of ambient temperature on the thermal balance of the body. The passive defence is the thermal inertia of brain and body which is sufficient to buffer transient thermal imbalances due to sleep processes. In addition, under the influence of heavy thermal loads and in the presence of an important pressure for sleep (Parmeggiani, 1987), autonomic temperature regulation is activated during NREM sleep without eliciting immediate awakening from sleep. This defence is energetically more costly; but as a consequence of the maintenance of brain thermal homeostasis, REM sleep onset may also be promoted and sustained thanks to the thermal inertia of the brain. Furthermore, the more behavioural temperature regulation constrains the activation of autonomic temperature regulation the more it prevents awakening from sleep. Awakening is the ultimate active defence of brain homeothermy but at the expense primarily of REM sleep and secondarily of NREM sleep.

Defence of Brain's Blood Supply in Sleep

The supply of blood to the brain in NREM sleep presents no problems from the viewpoint of systemic homeostasis: it decreases according to the controlled decrease in metabolic activity. In contrast, both morphological and functional factors underlie the complex mechanism of the compartmentalised and specific defence of brain blood supply in REM sleep. This homeostatic response is not elicited by the integrative cardiovascular control exerted by the central neural commands. It is also characterised by a thermal epiphenomenon, consisting of the small increase in hypothalamic temperature during REM sleep that was discussed in the previous paragraph.

This increase, amounting to a few tenths of a degree Celsius at most, may appear of little physiological importance from a physicochemical viewpoint. Notwithstanding this conclusion, the study of the underlying mechanism has revealed that it is the key to understand why an adequate arterial blood flow to the brain is maintained in spite of the systemic circulatory disturbances in REM sleep.

Three major factors possibly underlie this brain temperature increase, during REM sleep: (i) the metabolic heat production of the nervous tissue; (ii) the arterial blood flow and (iii) the arterial blood temperature. The experimental evidence shows that the proximate causes of the rise in brain temperature related to REM sleep are practically two. Namely, the occurrence of a quantitative shift from a carotid blood supply to a vertebral blood supply to the circle of Willis and a depression of systemic (pinna of the ear and nasal mucosa) and selective brain cooling (countercurrent or conductive heat loss). The remote cause of the rise in brain temperature is the systemic hemodynamic alteration in REM sleep. The instability of autonomic cardiovascular regulation decreasing the cardiac output brings about a reduction of common carotid artery blood supplying the brain and the systemic heat exchangers of the head. This reduction, which depresses both systemic and selective brain cooling, is counterbalanced by blood flowing to the brain primarily from the vertebral arteries in the species (cat and rabbit) considered in this case.

Now in more detail, many studies have suggested various factors directly underlying the REM sleep-related increase in brain temperature (see Parmeggiani, 1980b). In particular, an increase in the metabolic heat production of the nervous tissue has been proposed by several authors (Delgado and Hanai, 1966; Kawamura and Sawyer, 1965; Kawamura *et al.*, 1966; Satoh, 1968; Tachibana, 1969). Other authors suggested as the main factor either the arterial blood flow (Dufour and Court, 1977; Kanzow *et al.*, 1962; Reivich, 1972; Risberg and Ingvar, 1973; Seylaz *et al.*, 1971; Shapiro and Rosendorff, 1975; Tachibana, 1969) or the arterial blood temperature (Baker and Hayward, 1967a,b; Hayward and Baker, 1969).

Considering all these proposals in the context of recent experimental evidence, the following conclusion is justified: the metabolic heat production of the nervous tissue appears to be an unlikely candidate as the primary cause of the observed change in brain temperature. In fact, several studies show that both brain metabolic rate and arterial blood flow increase in REM sleep with respect to NREM sleep (see Franzini, 1992; Maquet, 2000). On this basis, the increase in brain metabolic heat production is indirectly related to the rise in heat clearance by the increase in arterial blood flow. Therefore, temperature alone is not a reliable indicator of changes in metabolic heat production (Hayward and Baker, 1969; Serota, 1939; Serota and Gerard, 1938). In any case, metabolic heat production is unlikely to play a major role in the increase of brain temperature related to REM sleep, a conclusion based on the experimental evidence presented below.

The other factors to be considered are the flow and the temperature of the arterial blood supplied to the circle of Willis by different sources. The effects of a transient fall in common carotid blood flow were studied in cats and rabbits (Azzaroni and Parmeggiani, 1993; Parmeggiani *et al.*, 2002). The fall was provoked by short (≤100s), bilateral common carotid artery occlusion during wakefulness and NREM sleep at ambient temperature (25 ± 2°C), close to thermal neutrality of these species. A decrease in ear pinna temperature and an increase in both preoptic-hypothalamic and pontine temperatures were elicited by this procedure. Different mechanisms underlie these temperature changes. The short latency and the steepness of the initial rise in preoptic-hypothalamic temperature appear to be an obvious effect of brain autoregulation of blood flow. The term autoregulation refers to both vascular and chemical mechanisms adjusting arterial blood flow to the metabolic rate of the nervous tissue (see Busija and Heistad, 1984). The metabolic demand of the cerebral bed, deprived by the fall in the carotid artery's share of cerebral blood flow, buffers the fall in carotid blood supply by increasing the supply of vertebral artery blood. The flow increase in vertebral artery blood, warmer (systemic cooling only) than carotid artery blood (both systemic and selective cooling), initially contributes more to the increase in preoptic-hypothalamic temperature than the depression of selective brain cooling. This temperature approaches but does not reach the also rising value of the pontine temperature during the short duration of bilateral common carotid artery occlusion. The pontine temperature rises with a lesser slope than preoptic-hypothalamic temperature, driven by the slower increase in temperature of vertebral artery blood (systemic cooling only) due to the large thermal inertia of the body. The latter rise is a result of the decrease in common carotid artery's blood flow, which depresses systemic heat loss from upper airway mucosa and the pinna of the ear. It is worth mentioning that electroencephalographic signs of ischemia are absent during bilateral common carotid artery occlusion of long (up to 300s) but evidently harmless duration in cats (Azzaroni and Parmeggiani, 1993). In this case, the preoptic-hypothalamic and pontine temperatures tend to plateau following the initial rise. This is a sign of the new thermal equilibrium existing between metabolic heat production and decreased systemic and selective heat loss.

Returning now to the issue of this section of the chapter, that is, the defence of the brain's blood supply in REM sleep, additional experimental evidence shows that the previous arguments also apply to the spontaneous increase in preoptic-hypothalamic and pontine temperatures related to this sleep state (Azzaroni and Parmeggiani, 1993; Parmeggiani *et al.*, 2002). This increase is characterised initially by a rather steep slope from the level attained at the end of NREM sleep and subsequently by a plateau. The temperature plateau lasts for the duration of the REM sleep episode and shows only small oscillations opposite to those of ear pinna temperature resulting in small changes of the systemic heat loss.

Bilateral, short (≤100s) occlusion of the common carotid artery at REM sleep onset in cats and rabbits does not affect, or only scarcely enhances, the spontaneous decrease in ear pinna temperature and the spontaneous increase in both preoptic-hypothalamic and pontine temperatures. This is a crucial result demonstrating that common carotid blood flow is spontaneously decreased on REM sleep occurrence. This decrease may be considered the trigger for an autoregulatory response increasing brain blood flow in REM sleep. There is experimental evidence in the cat that the spontaneous increase in hypothalamic blood flow during REM sleep is preceded by an initial transient decrease (Denoyer *et al.*, 1992; Roussel and Bittel, 1979; Roussel *et al.*, 1980). On this basis, the conclusion is warranted that bilateral occlusion of the common carotid artery in wakefulness and NREM sleep mimics a hemodynamic condition occurring spontaneously in REM sleep. In contrast, short bilateral common carotid artery occlusion after the end of REM sleep stops both the spontaneous increase in ear pinna temperature and the spontaneous decrease in pontine and preoptic-hypothalamic temperatures. This shows that common carotid artery blood flow spontaneously increases after the end of REM sleep: the increase enhances both systemic and selective brain cooling in turn; whereas vertebral artery blood flow decreases. The indirect experimental evidence of a spontaneous fall and rise in common carotid artery blood flow during and after REM sleep, respectively, has been confirmed by direct measurement of this flow in rabbits as shown in the following table (Calasso and Parmeggiani, 2008). Table 4 presents the changes in cardiovascular variables across wake–sleep states.

As mentioned before, preoptic-hypothalamic temperature rises during REM sleep also at low ambient temperature (Alföldi *et al.*, 1990; Franzini *et al.*, 1982; Parmeggiani *et al.*, 1971, 1975, 1977, 1984). The event is fairly inconsistent with the actual increased heat loss due to paradoxical vasodilatation of the systemic heat exchangers of the head (pinna of the ear, upper

Table 4. Carotid blood flow and heart rate during the ultradian sleep states (rabbit). Carotid mean flow and peak flow, and heart rate decrease in REMS with respect to NREMS. On arousing from REM sleep (wake), such variables increase with a steep slope above NREMS values. The data are presented as mean ± SEM. The variations of the mean values of the cardiovascular variables across epochs are statistically significant (Wilcoxon matched-pairs test, 5 pairs significance level: $P < 0.05$) with the exception of the difference of peak flow from REMS1 to REMS2. NREMS, NREM sleep; REMS, REM sleep: first half (1) and second half (2) of the episode. WAKE, arousing from sleep. (Data from Calasso and Parmeggiani, 2008.)

State	Carotid mean flow, ml/min	Carotid peak flow, ml/min	Heart rate, beats/min
NREMS	44.66 ± 1.05	118.99 ± 7.42	169.62 ± 2.42
REMS1	35.91 ± 1.37	94.06 ± 4.40	158.63 ± 1.77
REMS2	36.84 ± 1.28	92.35 ± 3.56	162.54 ± 2.01
WAKE	49.81 ± 1.20	126.49 ± 6.73	180.58 ± 2.07

airway mucosa) as mentioned in Chapter 5. This fact adds further indirect evidence that autoregulation of brain blood flow in REM sleep counterbalances the decrease in carotid blood supply to the brain by the increase in vertebral blood supply that is warmer (only systemic cooling) than the former (systemic and selective cooling).

The hemodynamic mechanisms described apply not only to cats and rabbits but probably also to rats that show comparable REM sleep-related changes of upper airway mucosa, preoptic-hypothalamic and pontine temperatures (Calasso and Parmeggiani, 2004; Calasso *et al.*, 1993). On the other hand, the internal carotid arteries are much larger than the vertebral arteries in primates (Edvinsson *et al.*, 1993). This difference underlies the unfavourable hemodynamic conditions, particularly in humans (Hale, 1960), for a significant enhancement of the blood supply of the vertebral arteries to the brain during REM sleep. Although the lack of adequate experimental evidence precludes any definitive conclusion, it is probable that brain temperature changes in primates depend mainly on changes in systemic brain cooling during REM sleep as a result of the large prevalence of carotid blood flow with respect to vertebral blood flow.

Systemic Functional Implications

The changes in blood flow of the common carotid and vertebral arteries revealed by the previous experimental results explain in detail the mechanism underlying the REM sleep-related rise in preoptic-hypothalamic temperature in cats, rabbits and rats. However, it should not be overlooked that the decrease in common carotid artery blood flow characterising REM sleep (Calasso and Parmeggiani, 2008) is the result of a systemic hemodynamic depression that appears so conspicuous as to affect negatively also vertebral artery blood flow and, consequently, cerebral autoregulation. However, an increase in cerebral blood flow during REM sleep with respect to NREM sleep was observed in several species including the cat and rabbit (see Franzini, 1992, 2005; Maquet, 2000). Therefore, a basic question is how to reconcile the systemic hemodynamic depression in REM sleep with the autoregulatory increase in cerebral blood flow. This is conceptually possible considering the factors that may contribute to an adequate autoregulation (both vascular and metabolic) of cerebral blood flow in spite of systemic unfavourable hemodynamic circumstances. The anatomical data (see Edvinsson *et al.*, 1993) point to important morphofunctional differences between the carotid and vertebral tributaries of the circle of Willis in the species considered. The differences are the complex network of fine vessels of the carotid rete in the cat and the vertebral arteries larger than the internal carotid arteries in the rabbit. On this basis, higher inflow impedance for the carotid blood supply than for the vertebral blood supply to the circle of Willis is likely in both cats and rabbits. In this respect, the disappearance of the negative hydrostatic load as a result of the lowered head posture, and a decrease in cerebral vascular impedance in relation with cortical activation in REM sleep also deserve consideration. The increase in the vertebral blood supply to the brain in the rabbit during REM sleep is also suggested by the fact that arterial blood flow increases more in the hindbrain than in the forebrain (see Franzini, 1992).

The autoregulatory response to the decreased common carotid artery blood supply to the forebrain is a result of the alteration of homeostatic cardiovascular regulation during REM sleep (see Franzini, 2005; Parmeggiani, 1994). However, an additional autoregulatory increase in vertebral blood supply is likely to occur as a response to the metabolic request of brain activation in REM sleep with respect to NREM sleep. The former autoregulatory response is the most variable, since the reduction of common carotid artery blood is due to autonomic events that are intrinsically irregular. The latter autoregulatory response is the most stable as the expression of actual flow-metabolism coupling due to the stereotyped pattern of brain activation in REM sleep. Eventually, the overall temporal coupling of flow and metabolism in the brain is less consistent in REM sleep than in both wakefulness and NREM sleep, according to the different time courses of randomly interacting peripheral and central physiological processes during REM sleep.

Conclusion

The mechanisms maintaining the temperature and the arterial blood flow of the brain within homeostatic limits during the ultradian sleep cycle are strictly interconnected. This statement conceals a very complex and baffling physiological reality that cannot be approached by sheer simplification. The effort to systematise and generalise the physiological mechanisms of homeostasis ought to respect the great variety of "amazing" solutions sustaining life in many different forms. Therefore, we may agree with Feyerabend's opinion that "*anything goes*" (Feyerabend, 1975) if it has been successfully tested throughout phylogeny.

Chapter 8

Ultradian Homeostasis–Poikilostasis Cycle

In the previous chapters, the physiological phenomenology characterising homeostasis and poikilostasis has been dissected in relation to the states of the ultradian sleep cycle. This chapter deals in general with the behavioural effects of the evolution of neural mechanisms for physiological homeostasis in mammals, based on the concept of a behavioural activity–rest cycle as the primitive expression of the neural control of the catabolic–anabolic balance of the living organism. A cycle with evolutionary implications as originally pointed out by Kleitman (see Kleitman, 1963).

From the procedural viewpoint of analysis, study of the changes in the regulation of the different physiological functions across the behavioural continuum is necessary to determine whether a systemic homeostasis–poikilostasis cycle exists underlying the differentiation of the behavioural states. In other words, the issue is essentially the nature of the neural control of the wake–sleep behaviour of mammals in response to the several endogenous and exogenous cues that challenge physiological homeostasis.

According to the criteria outlined in Chapter 2, this study takes into consideration particularly the systemic physiological operators of the somatic and autonomic mechanisms underlying homeostasis. Only continuous adjustments of the activity of these operators can meet successfully the predictable and unpredictable challenges arising within and without the organism by keeping the oscillations of the physiological parameters within the "normal" range of their values. This range, which depends on changes in the set point of the control mechanisms in wakefulness and NREM sleep, is also under the influence of circadian pacemakers. On the contrary, REM sleep is characterised by a disintegrated and disordered activity of many physiological operators resulting from the lack of a precise and stable integrative neural control. In this case, the major safety factor for the organism against dangerous quantitative drifts of physiological parameters appears to be the short duration of the REM sleep episode. The episode is differently modulated in duration in reciprocal relationship with the surface-to-volume ratio of various species (e.g., rats, rabbits, cats, humans) as well as by several ambient and organic conditions (temperature, light, darkness, body mass, fur, nutrition, predator or prey, etc.). Arousal from REM sleep normally limits its duration before there are endangering changes in the physiological parameters.

Ultradian Homeostasis–Poikilostasis Cycle

The ultradian wake–sleep cycle is characterised by three modalities of neural regulation of physiological functions, two being homeostatic and one poikilostatic.

Predictive homeostasis involves physiological changes due to exogenous or endogenous cues influencing ultradian and circadian pacemakers. The resulting anticipatory and progressive adjustments of the physiological functions are not immediately homeostatic in operation as in the case of reactive homeostasis. Substantially, predictive homeostasis improves the effectiveness of the reactive homeostatic defence of the organism. For instance, as far as thermoregulation is concerned there are seasonal variations of the layer of subcutaneous fat, thickness of fur, nutritional habits. Reactive homeostasis, in turn, encompasses all physiological responses to external ambient and internal disturbances influencing directly or indirectly the physiological parameters. Predictive and reactive homeostasis are operative in wakefulness and in NREM sleep, and suspended (poikilostasis) in REM sleep. However, the positive influence of predictive homeostasis on sleep is not completely lost in REM sleep as shown, e.g., by the passively maintained sleep postures and ecological niches.

Behavioural Expression of the Ultradian Homeostasis–Poikilostasis Cycle

The behavioural epoch including wakefulness and NREM sleep, which is characterised by homeostatic regulation, may be considered as an advanced phylogenetic expression of a basic catabolic–anabolic cycle. The presence and persistence of homeostatic regulation in this epoch is associated with the great development of the central nervous system in mammals. In particular, the specific operative logic of the neural control of homeostasis is common to both behavioural states. The main difference consists in the homeostatic demand of the prevailing relationship either with the environment or with the organism, that is expressed by an observable dynamic behaviour in wakefulness and is not obvious in the observable static behaviour in NREM sleep. From the physiological point of view both states are the result of the integrated goal-directed activity of somatic and autonomic mechanisms brought about by the homeostatic neural control substantially characterised by closed-loop operations. Wakefulness and NREM sleep, therefore, can be considered as being at the opposite ends of an intensity continuum of homeostatic regulation with maximum and minimum of metabolic rate, maximum and minimum of body temperature, sympathetic and parasympathetic reciprocal prevalence, etc. The operative logic of the neural control of both behavioural states is different only in quantitative terms, but still consistent with the qualitative functional criterion of the integrated control of homeostasis.

Between the subsequent cycles of this natural sequence of activity and rest occurring under the protecting shield of physiological homeostasis, there is the almost sudden intrusion of an epoch of poikilostatic physiological control. Normally, this intrusion occurs in NREM sleep, that is, in a condition of lowered metabolic rate. Premonitory signs are often a small decrease in hypothalamic temperature in cats and rats (Azzaroni and Parmeggiani, 1995b; Capitani et al., 2005; Parmeggiani et al., 1975), a decrease in delta and an increase in theta and sigma EEG power values in rats (Capitani et al., 2005). However, such changes maximally predict only 60% of the successful transitions from NREM to REM sleep in rats (Capitani et al., 2005). To this effect, there are other promoting conditions in NREM sleep, e.g., safe ecological niche, ambient thermal neutrality, and in particular, autonomic (sympathetic) quiescence (Azzaroni and Parmeggiani, 1995b). They are relevant to REM sleep occurrence particularly in the absence of a debt of REM sleep due to deprivation for one reason or another. Otherwise, the existence of a debt may force the breakthrough of REM sleep under less favourable ambient thermal conditions than thermal neutrality (Amici *et al.*, 1994, 1998; Cerri *et al.*, 2005; Parmeggiani and Rabini, 1970; Parmeggiani *et al.*, 1980). The more the physiological equilibrium between environment and organism is maintained at low metabolic rate in NREM sleep, the less the occurrence of the typical physiological phenomena of REM sleep is obliterated by a prompt arousal from sleep.

The daily need for NREM sleep is measurable quantitatively by the "intensity" of the EEG power density in the delta band (0.75–4 Hz). According to the two-process model (see Borbely and Achermann, 2005), this intensity is the expression of the process S that quantifies the intrinsic sleep need showing an increase during wakefulness. The other process is the circadian regulation of sleep propensity (process C) underlying the distribution of sleep during the 24 hours in the different species preferably according to endogenous and exogenous conditions favouring ecological safety, nutrition, energy saving and physiological homeostasis. The exponential decay of the increased power density to the normal power density in the delta band does not require a particularly long time to occur both in humans (see Borbély and Achermann, 2005) and rats (Cerri *et al.*, 2005). The debt of NREM sleep is therefore more easily paid as a result of the practical absence of the additional quantitative temporal constraint of a conspicuous obligatory daily duration that is typical of REM sleep. The basic dynamical difference of the two recovery processes depends on the exponential intensity decay of the NREM sleep debt after deprivation and the linear temporal decay of the REM sleep debt after deprivation. In the latter case the time required for the recovery from the debt is directly proportional to the debt itself in addition to the obligatory daily quota of REM sleep (Parmeggiani and Rabini, 1970; Parmeggiani *et al.*, 1980).

The quantitative analysis of short-term deprivation and recovery of REM sleep in cats exposed to low ambient temperature (−10°C) has shown that the accumulation of the REM sleep debt is a fairly continuous process developing during day and night. Nevertheless, the payment of the debt after return to neutral ambient temperature is a discontinuous process included in the ultradian cycle of sleep. The recovery of the lost REM sleep develops with episodes of increased frequency but variable duration depending on the amount of the debt itself and the circadian modulation of sleep under the influence of ambient and organic factors (Parmeggiani *et al.*, 1980). In the rat, the recovery of REM sleep debt after deprivation at low ambient temperature (−10°C), occurs at high rate (prevalence of sequential episodes) but only partially in the first day after return to neutral ambient temperature, and requires up to 4 days to be fully paid (Amici *et al.*, 2008). In conclusion, the expression of REM sleep is temporally limited and easily obliterated not only by the specific request of homeostatic regulation but also by multifarious changes in the level of vigilance under the influence of adverse organic and ambient conditions.

The need for a daily amount of REM sleep, revealed by the effects of deprivation, appears to be an important timing factor underlying the temporal structure of the ultradian cycle of sleep. The necessary daily cumulative duration of REM sleep is normally achieved by changes in the frequency and/or the duration of the episodes to compensate for temporal losses induced by endogenous and exogenous disturbing influences. Particularly interesting in this respect is the positive correlation of the duration of the REM sleep episode with the duration of the following REM sleep free interval, including NREM sleep, before the next REM sleep episode (Amici *et al.*, 2008; Barbato and Wehr, 1998; Benington and Heller, 1994; Ursin, 1970; Vivaldi *et al.*, 1994). This fact shows that REM sleep duration influences the structure of both ultradian and circadian wake–sleep cycles. REM sleep is, therefore, a critical physiological event in the structure of sleep, pointing out the physiological necessity of the functional anarchy of systemic poikilostasis.

The utility of states like wakefulness and NREM sleep, as behavioural expressions of predictive and reactive homeostasis in response to organic and ambient challenges, is self-evident. The nature of the physiological need of a switch toward poikilostasis, however, is still the object of hypotheses that will be considered later. Now, only the question of whether the sequence of sleep events might be also the result of a genetic determination of the ultradian homeostasis–poikilostasis-cycle will be taken into detailed consideration.

Sleep and Instinct

The study of the somatic and autonomic physiology of wakefulness and NREM sleep shows that their regulation paradigms perfectly meet the requirements of a balanced interaction between environment and organism in the temporal continuum of life. The systemic homeostatic control of bodily functions in either activity or rest is, therefore, the result of the same operative logic but at different rates of energy expenditure. A true functional dichotomy exists, instead, between NREM and REM sleep. In the latter, the effects of open-loop processes of central neural origin, also altering feedback controls, bring about the suppression or depression of the integrated reactive homeostasis. Since poikilostasis normally emerges in mammals only during sleep from the background of efficient autonomic mechanisms for physiological homeostasis, there may be a relationship between this basic homeostasis–poikilostasis cycle and the phylogenetic evolution of sleep states.

In this context, poikilostasis may be considered the dramatic but regulated expression of a basic and still mysterious functional need of the nervous system. A need, which is possible to cope with only during a behavioural state resulting virtually from the functional hierarchical inversion of the course of the phylogenesis, that provided the hierarchical morphological and functional organisation of the central nervous system in mammals. This inverse course of sleep is so deeply rooted in the physiology of mammals as to appear genetically determined. In this respect, the issue deserves to be examined briefly to see whether there is a clear indication of the instinctive nature of the homeostasis–poikilostasis cycle underlying sleep behaviour as actually determined by the systemic neural control.

After the pioneering approach by Claparède (1905) to the instinctive nature of sleep, the work of ethologists, in particular, has shown many instinctive aspects of sleep behaviour. For example, Tinbergen (1951, p. 112) defines an instinct as "*a hierarchically organised nervous mechanism which is susceptible to certain priming, releasing and directing impulses of internal as well as external origin, and which responds to these impulses by coordinated movements that contribute to the maintenance of the individual and the species.*"

In particular, according to ethologists (see Craig, 1918; Hediger, 1959, 1969; Hinde, 1966; Holzapfel, 1940; Lashley, 1938; Lorenz, 1956; Tinbergen, 1951) an instinct must present the several essential qualifications that are listed as follows. (i) Complex pattern of sensory-motor integration and neural hierarchical organisation. (ii) Appetitive behaviour modifiable by learning while the consummatory act is innate. (iii) Instability of the appetitive phase and stability of the consummatory phase. (iv) Typical changes in physiological functions. (v) Satiation after the consummatory act as a self-inhibitory effect. (vi) Necessity for preservation of the individual and the species. (vii) Actively produced and determined by internal and external factors. (viii) Not necessarily bound to motor activity.

The study of the neurophysiology of sleep has also shown that this behaviour meets such qualifications (Moruzzi, 1969; Parmeggiani, 1968).

The operative model of instinctive activity points out the basic importance of the *"consummatory act"*. Particularly, the precise identification of such an act is the basis for considering sleep behaviour to be the biological expression of an instinct. However, sleep reveals no clear-cut physiological and behavioural features of the occurrence of a consummatory act as it is normally recognised with wakefulness. This is a clear difference between sleep and classical instinctive patterns characterised by manifest consummatory acts, such as eating or mating. However, it is worth considering that, if the consummatory act of sleep is a process effected within the nervous system as an internal event, it may not show an obvious behavioural pattern of somatic and autonomic interaction with the environment. To support this possibility also in the case of sleep behaviour, two fundamental properties of the consummatory act ought to be verified. Firstly, that it is a physiologically compulsory process, and secondly, that it may be defined not only in qualitative but also in quantitative terms. According to these criteria, a consistent expression of an endogenous need of the central nervous system may be considered when considering the occurrence of REM sleep (Parmeggiani, 1973). One thinks of two reasons for this conclusion. The first is that the process is physiologically important, particularly because the autonomic thermoregulation, a specific and fundamental function in mammals, is suspended. The second is that the process is necessary on a quantitative temporal basis as shown by the effects of its temperature-dependent deprivation and recovery, which has already been considered in more detail (see Chapters 5 and 6). Thus, REM sleep appears to be the best candidate for the role of consummatory act (Parmeggiani, 1968, 1973). On the other hand, the precise homeostatic regulation of physiological activity characterising NREM sleep appears consistent with an appetitive (predictive) state controlling the occurrence of a consummatory act basically altering homeostatic regulation in mammals.

In addition to these considerations, it is most important to mention genetic studies of sleep behaviour. Using inbred strains of mice and their crossing, workers demonstrated that the hereditary component is important not only for the determination of sleep but also for the duration and the circadian rhythmicity of each state (Valatx *et al.*, 1972; Valatx and Bugat, 1974). In recent years, moreover, the genetic study of sleep in *Drosophila melanogaster* has shown that its regulation involves several genes, a result again supporting the concept of the instinctive nature of sleep (Huber *et al.*, 2004).

Functional Significance of Homeostasis and Poikilostasis in Sleep

As will be discussed below, the changes in the modality of physiological regulation during sleep with respect to wakefulness involve not only adaptation to the environment, but also basic functional needs of the organism.

In general, the restriction of catabolic energy expenditure surely has a high survival value. This criterion applies particularly to NREM sleep. In REM sleep, however, the increase in the metabolic rate of the brain is associated with the surrender of the homeostatic regulation of physiological functions. As a result of the homeostasis–poikilostasis switch (see Chapter 2), the bimodal neural control of physiological functions is the fundamental marker of the basically different physiology of the two sleep states. In particular, the study of the interaction between thermoregulatory, respiratory, cardiovascular functions on the one side and sleep states on the other has revealed a number of systemic physiological phenomena showing a consistency which has stood the test of time.

In active wakefulness, the changes in the regulation of physiological operators are the result of volitional and instinctive drives sometimes overwhelming, but only temporarily, homeostatic neural regulation. The physiological purpose of such events is clear in this behavioural state, characterised by the active interaction of the organism with the environment. On the contrary, the homeostatic states of functional rest, as in quiet wakefulness and NREM sleep, appear as recovery periods under the tight homeostatic control of the central nervous system over the body.

Still a question mark is the poikilostatic condition of REM sleep in the adult mammal, precisely because it is equipped with a precise control of physiological functions. A possible answer to this question is suggested by the way chosen by *Nature* to integrate, in the sequential behavioural frame of the sleep cycle, two opposite organisations of physiological regulation, first the one of more advanced (homeostatic) design and then the other of more primitive (poikilostatic) design. The full expression of the neuronal activity of the primitive brain stem level (medulla and pons) is, however, partially hidden at the somatic level by the atonia of skeletal muscles. The change from homeostatic to poikilostatic regulation during the ultradian sleep cycle may be considered as a process of separate tuning of the activity of different neuronal networks, organised in series and in parallel at different hierarchical levels in the brain stem. The open-loop mode of physiological regulation in REM sleep may restore the efficiency of the different neuronal networks of the brain stem by expressing also genetically coded patterns of instinctive behaviour that are kept normally hidden from view by skeletal muscle atonia. Such behaviourally concealed neuronal activity was demonstrated by the effects of experimental lesions of specific pontine structures (Hendricks, 1982; Hendricks *et al.*, 1977, 1982; Henley and Morrison, 1974; Jouvet and Delorme, 1965; Sastre and Jouvet, 1979; Villablanca, 1966). Not only was the skeletal muscle atonia suppressed but also motor fragments of complex instinctive behaviours appeared, such as walking and attack, that were not externally motivated (see Morrison, 2005). These experimental results, together with the normal manifestation of electroencephalographic desynchronisation, skeletal muscle twitches and jerks and ponto-geniculo-occipital waves point to an endogenous process of neuronal activation in REM sleep.

Study of the organisation of the highly integrated thermoregulatory mechanisms in mammals demonstrates in general what might functionally occur during REM sleep. The anatomical basis of this inference is that all the steps of the morphofunctional evolution of the mechanisms of thermoregulation in the course of phylogenesis are preserved in hierarchical order of appearance in the structures of the neuraxis (see Satinoff, 1978). In the abstract, this organisation may be considered a modular structure.

The activity of such modules, that are not independent of each other, is facilitated or inhibited by those that are placed more cranially in the brain stem. The role of the hypothalamus in this complex network of thermoregulatory mechanisms placed at different levels of the neuraxis is only the most important because it coordinates their set points of activation. Similarly, study of respiration and circulation shows that their basic control mechanisms at pontine and medullary levels are hierarchically coordinated in hypothalamic and telencephalic structures (e.g., amygdala, orbital frontal cortex) during wakefulness and NREM sleep. In REM sleep, this hierarchical coordination of different mechanisms ceases and a state of functional open-loop anarchy develops.

A physiological hypothesis for the teleological significance of homeostasis in active and quiet wakefulness is clearly less daring and more straightforward than in the case of NREM sleep and REM sleep. Active and quiet wakefulness may be considered the expressions of the homeostatic catabolic and anabolic extremes of the behavioural relationship of the organism with the environment. What appears from the neurophysiological viewpoint in NREM sleep and REM sleep suggests that these states may be the expressions of a genetically determined process of neural autoregulation, a resetting of brain functions requiring a restriction of the energetic demands of other physiological functions of the body in favour of the nervous system.

Of the several hypotheses concerning the functional significance of sleep, only one is considered here, since it appears the most adequate and general to explain the basic issue of this book. Accordingly, it is possible that a general and basic function of sleep may be related to the functional recovery of synapses according to the *"synaptic homeostasis hypothesis"* (see Tononi and Cirelli, 2005). This hypothesis argues that sleep processes play a role in the regulation of the synaptic weight in the brain, being involved in morphologic and metabolic synaptic downscaling in order to eliminate the selective synaptic potentiation occurring in wakefulness. Wakefulness is characterised by long-term potentiation in many cortical circuits producing a net increase in their synaptic weight. Therefore, a general synaptic downscaling during sleep contributes to maintenance of a balanced synaptic input to all cortical neurons. This process may be revealed in NREM sleep by slow-wave electroencephalographic activity. According to this hypothesis, the rhythmical and synchronised activity of thalamic and cortical neurons underlying slow waves would promote a generalised depression or down-scaling of synapses in the telencephalon. Neuronal plasticity would be recovered as a result of such general synaptic downscaling. In contrast to NREM sleep, downscaling of synapses would be produced in REM sleep by random bursts of neuronal firing (e.g., also bursts underlying ponto-geniculo-occipital waves) (see Tononi and Cirelli, 2005).

This hypothesis is particularly enriched in functional significance by considering at this point the opposite nature, homeostatic and poikilostatic, of the systemic neural regulation of physiological functions in these sleep states. The important fact is that homeostasis is fully preserved in NREM sleep. This means that a systemic synaptic downscaling (slow-wave elec-troencephalographic activity) is practically limited to the relatively homogeneous cortical structures of the telencephalon, while the whole brain stem, from diencephalon to medulla, is still exerting its basic func-tions of integrated homeostatic regulation of both somatic and autonomic physiological functions. In REM sleep, however, the necessary synaptic downscaling in the brain stem is instead a result of random neuronal firing. This fact shows that the neuronal circuitry of the brain stem is functionally disassembled and therefore active in an apparently disorderly fashion that brings about the poikilostatic control of autonomic physiological functions in particular. This anarchical brain stem activation is also reflected in the endogenous desynchronisation of the electroencephalogram, a sort of arousal in sleep lacking significant environmental inputs and therefore underlying dreaming consciousness.

To sum up, the physiological necessity of poikilostasis in REM sleep is worth being stressed. The functional plasticity of the neuronal net-works at the different levels of the complex hierarchical organisation of the brain stem may be particularly weakened during the tonic closed-loop homeostatic control of the physiological parameters that is carried out in wakefulness and in NREM sleep. In this respect, it is also interesting to add that in REM sleep there is even the cessation of activity in the aminergic neurons to prevent desensitisation of aminergic receptors, which are con-tinuously activated in waking (Siegel and Rogawsky, 1988). Skeletal muscle atonia that avoids potential behavioural inadequacy to environmental dan-gers is important for the recovery of the normal functional plasticity and of steadily inhibited genetically coded patterns of instinctive behaviour. According to this way of thinking, REM sleep is the physiological expression of the partially hidden neural mechanisms underlying the ultimate functional significance of poikilostasis as a restoring process of brain stem functional efficiency.

Conclusion

The usefulness of the principle of homeostasis as a criterion for differentiating the states of sleep in terms of systemic physiological functions has been discussed on the basis of the experimental results presented in the previous chapters. This approach is motivated by the work of Cannon, who expressed confidence that *"homeostasis is not accidental but a result of organized government, and that search for the governing agencies will result in their discovery"* (1929, p. 426).

Theoretically, the principle easily fits the teleological aspect of systemic physiological regulation in positive (homeostasis) and negative (poikilostasis) terms. The identification of basic differences in the applicability of the principle to the behavioural states is a step in the discovery of still hidden "governing agencies". However, the interpretation of the experimental data, presented in this book, also shows how complex and articulated ought to be the search for the principle(s) underlying the different behavioural states. The ultimate difficulty depends on the fact that compartmentalised and auto-regulatory mechanisms underlying homeostasis may be mechanistically unrelated with the logic of the straightforward systemic homeostatic controls (e.g., see Chapter 7). It is therefore difficult to expand the scrutiny from the classical physiological realm of systemic functions beyond the boundaries worked out here. Another reason is that the distinction between physiological parameter and operator can be maintained only at systemic levels. This distinction is not operationally discriminative within the mechanistic complexity of molecular biology, since in this realm there is an almost inseparable parameter–operator dualism in the function of many variables (see Chapter 1).

Chapter 9

Systemic Physiological Regulation in the Ultradian Wake–Sleep Cycle

This chapter presents a model describing the changes in the functional organisation of the central nervous system during the ultradian wake–sleep cycle according to the observed physiological phenomena. The model is conceived from the perspective of both a morphological and a functional approach to the organisation of the central nervous system as brought about by phylogenetic and ontogenetic processes (Parmeggiani, 1982, 1985). The model compares the stable anatomical partition of the brain with its variable physiological activities that underlay the ultradian homeostasis–poikilostasis cycle of mammals. In other words, the changes in physiological regulation in the wake–sleep states are considered to be the result of hierarchical permutations in the functional organisation of major subdivisions of the encephalon (telencephalon, diencephalon and rhombencephalon). Current knowledge has revealed that the neural structures underlying the generation of NREM sleep are principally located in the diencephalon (anterior hypothalamus and adjacent forebrain, the latter actually being a part of the telencephalon) and of REM sleep in the rhombencephalon (pons).

Hierarchical Functional Permutations

The sequence of behavioural states starts with wakefulness and ends with REM sleep. The sequence *wake–sleep* is conventional but it is used in this book because its basic criterion of analysis is the hierarchical anatomical evolution of the encephalon. Sleep researchers prefer the inverse sequence

Table 5. The functional hierarchical array varies during the ultradian wake–sleep cycle, whereas the morphological hierarchical array is obviously invariant. MHA, morphological hierarchical array; FHA, functional hierarchical arrays; QW, quiet wakefulness; NREMS, NREM sleep; REMS, REM sleep; T, telencephalon; D, diencephalon; R, rhombencephalon. (Modified from Parmeggiani, 1982.)

MHA		FHA		
Rank		QW	NREMS	REMS
I	T	T	D	R
II	D	D	R	T
III	R	R	T	D

of *sleep–wake*, but this usage is more arbitrary than *wake–sleep* since sleep is emphasised as the object of primary interest.

In the model (Table 5), the behavioural states are considered the result of permutations in the functional dominance (>) of the major subdivisions of the encephalon. Three ranks of functional dominance (I > II > III) are variously given to the telencephalon (T), the diencephalon (D) and the rhombencephalon (R) for the various states on the basis of the physiological regulation of effector mechanisms. As a result, the functional hierarchical array varies during the ultradian wake–sleep cycle, whereas the morphological hierarchical array (T > D > R) is the obviously invariant reference. The transitions from wakefulness to sleep, and vice versa, and from NREM sleep to REM sleep occur due to the descent of the first rank structure to the third rank and the ascent in the functional influence of the second and third rank structures to the contiguous superior ranks.

Out of six theoretically possible permutations ($3 \times 2 \times 1 = 6$) in the hierarchical arrays of functional dominance, only three (T > D > R in wakefulness; D > R > T in NREM sleep; R > T > D in REM sleep) occur naturally in adult mammals. Such functional permutations in the central nervous system conform to the physiological phenomena observed during the normal ultradian wake–sleep cycle. The functional significance of the other three permutations (T > R > D, D > T > R, R > D > T) will be considered afterwards.

The limiting criterion underlying the three normally permitted permutations in the adult organism acknowledges the great stability of the diencephalic–rhombencephalic hierarchical and functional relationship (D > R), which is also inherent in the structural continuity of the diencephalic and rhombencephalic cores. This hierarchical relationship is strong and the basic condition for the development of the normal sequence of behavioural states of the ultradian wake–sleep cycle. Neither the hierarchical inversion (R > D) in a normal and undisturbed sleep cycle nor hierarchical splitting (D > T > R) occurs as a separate and durable event in normal conditions of sleep, that is in the absence of disturbing endogenous or exogenous influences. As a result, the hierarchical inversion of the diencephalic–rhombencephalic relationship is stable if it is associated with hierarchical splitting (R > T > D), revealed by the electroencephalographic desynchronisation in REM sleep. This condition (T in the II rank) does not correspond to a full arousal since the telencephalon is still under the control of REM sleep mechanisms.

The functional significance of the other three permutations (T > R > D, D > T > R, R > D > T) may apply to states of fetal and newborn normal or abnormal maturation of the central nervous system that will not be considered in this discussion. It is, however, interesting and pertinent to consider a particular case of the pathology of sleep in human adults, narcolepsy, since it involves this group of permutations of the hierarchical arrays of functional dominance. Narcolepsy is a chronic sleep disorder characterised by excessive daytime sleepiness and disturbed nocturnal sleep. There is an early intrusion of REM sleep and depression of NREM sleep in the ultradian sleep cycle. In this case, the permutations (T > R > D, D > T > R, R > D > T) deserve to be considered from a functional viewpoint. Concerning the array of wakefulness (T > R > D), the telencephalon loses the direct control of the diencephalon, which has descended to the lowest rank because the rhombencephalon gains in functional dominance over the diencephalon. The result is that the control system is much weaker and less stable than in normal wakefulness (T > D > R). With regard to the array of NREM sleep (D > T > R), the functional dominance of the diencephalon over the rhombencephalon is weakened by the interposition of the telencephalon, promoting further the instability of the control system with respect to normal NREM sleep (D > R > T). Concerning REM sleep, the

functional array (R > D > T) shows the dominance of the rhombencephalon over both diencephalon and telencephalon. The ultradian
sequences of these abnormal arrays are characterised by functional instability that randomly mixes phenomenal fragments of all wake–sleep states
as in cataplexy and other sleep disorders as parasomnias. Particularly
impressive is the phenomenon of cataplexy characterised by an abrupt loss
of muscle tone while awake.

From a general viewpoint, it is functionally significant to note that the
hierarchical controls are always only partially inverted in the normal ultradian sleep cycle with respect to wakefulness (T > D > R). The permutation
of NREM sleep (D > R > T) maintains the hierarchical control of the diencephalon over the rhombencephalon and the permutation of REM sleep
(R > T > D) maintains the hierarchical control of the telencephalon over
the diencephalon. In the first case, homeostasis is maintained during
NREM sleep, and in the second case of REM sleep, full wakefulness with
autonomic and somatic activation is almost immediately attainable. On the
contrary, in the case of the abnormal three permutations (T > R > D, D >
T > R, R > D > T) all normal hierarchical controls are totally lost.

In conclusion, the model is remarkably coherent with physiological and
pathological aspects of the ultradian wake–sleep cycle.

Influence of the Hierarchical Dynamics of the Ultradian Wake–Sleep Cycle on Physiological Functions

The transition from homeostasis to poikilostasis, and vice versa, may
be further pointed out via the hierarchical dynamics of the same model
(Fig. 15). As discussed above, the descent of the functional influence of the
first rank structure to the lowest rank (third) is associated with the ascent
of the second and third rank structures to the contiguous superior ranks
(first and second, respectively). In particular, two of the naturally occurring
ranks (in wakefulness and in NREM sleep) show the normal
diencephalic–rhombencephalic (D > R) hierarchical relationship (T > D >
R and D > R > T) and are both characterised by homeostatic regulation of
physiological functions. In contrast, the functional poikilostasis in REM
sleep depends on the loss of hierarchical coherence between the morphological (D > R) and the new functional organisation of the relationship

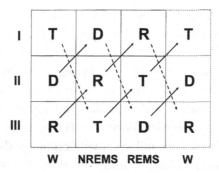

Fig. 15. Diagram showing the position in the ranks of functional dominance attained by the telencephalon (T), the diencephalon (D) and the rhombencephalon (R) in the states of wakefulness (W), NREM sleep (NREMS) and REM sleep (REMS). The array of structures in each behavioural state has been inferred from the changes in physiological regulation. The hierarchical permutations occur in an orderly way, as indicated by arrows. (Modified from Parmeggiani, 1982.)

between diencephalon and rhombencephalon (R > T > D). This is the result of the combined hierarchical split and inversion. Such a split, in addition to the functional dominance of the rhombencephalon, brings about the functional ascent of the telencephalon to the second rank and the descent of the diencephalon to the third rank. This new situation is functionally, characterised by the loss of homeostatic control and the desynchronisation of the electroencephalogram.

The proposed model stresses the critical function of diencephalic structures in the control of the somatic and autonomic phenomena of the ultradian wake–sleep cycle. In wakefulness, the telencephalic dominance (T > D > R) for the most adequate and versatile relationship of the organism to the ever-changing environment in terms of sensory–motor integration is sustained by the coincidence of the morphological and the functional hierarchical ranks of telencephalon, diencephalon and rhombencephalon. The model implies also that the transition from quiet wakefulness to NREM sleep (D > R > T) is rather smooth. No functional crisis occurs as a result of the maintained (D–R) hierarchical relationship. Moreover, during NREM sleep the maximum stability of automatic functions at a low transformation rate of energy is attained as a result of the lost functional dominance of telencephalic structures (D > R > T). In contrast, the hierarchical split and inversion (R > T > D) of the (D–R) functional relationship brings about a functional crisis at the rapid transition from NREM to REM sleep (homeostasis–poikilostasis switch). Evidently, this event has the highest probability of occurring when the (D–R) functional relationship is barely activated, that is, in conditions of thermal neutrality, and of basal metabolic, cardiovascular and respiratory activity. Any enhancement of the regulatory function of (D) opposes the (D) descent to the lowest hierarchical rank and eventually promotes the return of (T) to the first hierarchical rank and arousal from sleep. In contrast, the descent of (D) to the lowest hierarchical rank underlies the ascent of (R) to the first rank and REM sleep occurrence. The impaired hypothalamic homeostatic regulation in REM sleep, as a result of the loss of diencephalic dominance (R > T > D), releases neural mechanisms underlying a great instability of effector functions. However, this state is without dangerous behavioural consequences thanks to skeletal muscle atonia's impeding behavioural motor activity in a period of sleep still lacking the full awareness of the surrounding environment. The condition of functional instability is aggravated by the first step (ascent of T to the second rank) of telencephalic activation toward the first rank of wakefulness without the full functional support of awareness and homeostatic physiological control. The desynchronised EEG patterns may be considered a partial arousal in sleep (e.g., dream content with some logical structure) which differs substantially from a full arousal from any state of sleep.

In conclusion, the model points to the importance of interactive processes within the central nervous system broadly featuring the ultradian evolution of wake–sleep states in mammals as a stepwise, integrative regression. In a reverse fashion, the successive functional levels of the phylogenetic development of the encephalon are attained as the result of the functional loss of the hierarchical coherence between its morphological and physiological organisations. In other words, the three behavioural states may be considered separately as functional landmarks of the development of homeostatic mechanisms in the mammalian encephalon through successive superimposition of increasingly complex integrative levels.

Chapter 10

Epilogue

In the previous chapters evidence has been presented demonstrating that the ultradian sleep cycle is not determined by mere quantitative changes in the same modality of neural regulation, but rather consists of a sequence of two behavioural states characterised by qualitatively different paradigms of systemic physiological regulation.

In this respect, a remark concerning the current denomination of these states is appropriate from a semantic point of view. For example, the naming of a sleep state with an abstract term as "paradoxical" is not scientifically explicit, but rather it wittily reveals the surprise that a novel phenomenon of nature does not meet the previous theoretical inferences of sleep researchers. On the contrary, naming sleep states on the basis of a few concrete physiological phenomena (e.g., slow-eye-movement sleep and rapid-eye-movement sleep; synchronised sleep and desynchronised sleep) provides a practically acceptable but conceptually still partial definition. A few examples show the inadequacy of these definitions. The denomination of sleep stages on the basis of eye movements is more a remembrance of an historical discovery than indicative of basic changes in sleep physiology. Likewise, the electroencephalographic phenomenon of desynchronisation alone without analysis of the wave frequency, does not clearly distinguish wakefulness from REM sleep unless the electrogram of skeletal muscles is also considered. In short, all the appellations of states based only on a few characteristic phenomena are conceptually restrictive since they neglect many other important functional features of sleep.

On the basis of the data presented in the previous chapters, there is a reason to identify conceptually each behavioural state in accordance with the particular modality of systemic physiological regulation, either homeostatic or poikilostatic. Each modality may be conceived of as the abstract but stable link between the observed physiological phenomena and the activity of the neural mechanisms underlying their generation. In relation to the great number of different physiological events to be taken into account, the synthesising power of the concepts of homeostatic and poikilostatic regulation is remarkably consistent with the natural events of sleep. This consideration supports the opinion that a change in the labelling of sleep states would be convenient speaking practically and remarkably significant for its physiological implications. In other words, instead of focusing on only a few aspects of sleep phenomenology, the new definition of sleep states takes into account the global expression of the two modalities of neural regulation, that is to say, *homeostatic sleep and poikilostatic sleep*. In conclusion, the tenet of this book is that such basic changes in physiological regulation are also extrinsically expressed as whole sleep behaviours, a point of view that should be given serious consideration.

From the practical viewpoint of sleep medicine the two modalities of systemic physiological regulation in sleep clearly raise the question of an implicit physiological risk that foreshadows different pathological consequences (Parmeggiani, 1991). During sleep and particularly in poikilostatic sleep, a general factor of risk is the reduced repertory of adequate responses to harmful environmental influences in comparison with wakefulness, if arousal is ruled out as a first step of defence. Moreover, the risk differs in homeostatic sleep and poikilostatic sleep because of their specific modality of physiological regulation. In particular, the regulation by automatic physiological mechanisms in homeostatic sleep involves a risk mainly when they are altered by ageing or pathological organic conditions. Therefore, in conditions of good health the risk in homeostatic sleep may normally be considered as due to extrinsic causation, e.g., the threat of being predated or of pathological conditions. In contrast, the risk may be considered as intrinsic to poikilostatic sleep (although not exclusively) because of the suspension of integrative homeostatic regulation of physiological functions. Particularly this state may aggravate pathological conditions of respiration and circulation (e.g., sleep apnea or bradyarrhythmia). In response to such evidence, sleep medicine has rapidly progressed and branched into medical specialities concerning not only pure sleep disorders, but also psychiatric, neurological, respiratory and cardiovascular disorders, all related to the physiological basis of sleep (see Kryger *et al.*, 2005).

Besides the actual medical risks of sleep when pathological conditions are present, a basic biological issue is the teleological significance of taking a potential physiological risk in sleep and particularly in poikilostatic sleep. Up to now, the real nature of the biological necessity of the latter state is practically unknown. Of indisputable importance, however, is the surprising fact that the functional processes of poikilostatic sleep are a normal occurrence in the adult mammalian organism. Given that mammals are endowed by nature with a precise neural regulation of homeostasis, one may conclude that the presence of poikilostatic sleep is the behavioural expression of a basic functional need of the central nervous system itself. It is still a mysterious need that may involve, for instance, the restoration of noradrenergic receptor sensitivity (Siegel and Rogawsky, 1988), the homeostatic downscaling of the synaptic potentiation of wakefulness (see Tononi and Cirelli, 2005), memory processing (see Cipolli, 2005) or all three — and quite likely even more. These suggestions are the first important steps toward understanding the probably very complex nature of the function of sleep — a scientific conquest that will be a highlight not only of sleep research, but also of neuroscience in general.

References

Affanni, J.M., Lisogorsky, E. and Scaravilli, A.M. (1972). Sleep in the giant South American armadillo Priodontes giganteus (Edentata, Mammalia). *Experientia*, 28: 1046–1047.

Alam, M.N., McGinty, D. and Szymusiak R. (1995a). Neuronal discharge of preoptic/ anterior hypothalamic thermosensitive neurons: relation to NREM sleep. *Am. J. Physiol.*, 269: R1240–R1249.

Alam, M.N., McGinty, D. and Szymusiak, R. (1995b). Preoptic/anterior hypothalamic neurons: thermosensitivity in rapid eye movement sleep. *Am. J. Physiol.*, 269: R1250–R1257.

Alam, M.N., McGinty, D. and Szymusiak, R. (1997). Thermosensitive neurons of the diagonal band in rats: relation to wakefulness and non-rapid eye movement sleep. *Brain Res.*, 752: 81–89.

Alam, M.N., Gong, H., Alam, T., *et al.* (2002). Sleep–waking discharge patterns of neurons recorded in the rat perifornical lateral hypothalamic area. *J. Physiol.*, 538: 619–631.

Alföldi, P., Rubicsek, G., Cserni, G., *et al.* (1990). Brain and core temperatures and peripheral vasomotion during sleep and wakefulness at various ambient temperatures in the rat. *Pflügers Arch.*, 417: 336–341.

Altman, P.L. and Dittmer, D.S. (1966). *Environmental Biology*. Bethesda, MD: F.A.S.E.B.

Amici, R., Zamboni, G., Perez, E., *et al.* (1994). Pattern of desynchronised sleep during deprivation and recovery induced in the rat by changes in ambient temperature. *J. Sleep Res.*, 3: 250–256.

Amici, R., Zamboni, G., Perez, E., *et al.* (1998). The influence of a heavy thermal load on REM sleep in the rat. *Brain Res*, 781: 252–258.

Amici, R., Jones, C.A., Perez, E., *et al.* (2005). A physiological view of REM sleep structure. In: Parmeggiani, P.L. and Velluti, R. (eds), *The Physiologic Nature of Sleep*. London: Imperial College Press, 161–185.

Amici, R., Cerri, M., Ocampo-Garcés, A., *et al.* (2008). Cold exposure and sleep in the rat: REM sleep homeostasis and body size. *Sleep*, 31: 708–715.

Amoros, C., Sagot, J.C., Libert, J.P., *et al.* (1986). Sweat gland response to local heating during sleep in man. *J. Physiol.*, 81: 209–215.

Aserinsky, E. (1965). Periodic respiratory pattern occurring in conjunction with eye movements during sleep. *Science*, 150: 763–766.

Aserinsky, E. and Kleitman, N. (1953). Regularly occurring periods of eye motility and concomitant phenomena during sleep. *Science*, 118: 273–274.

Azzaroni, A. and Parmeggiani, P.L. (1993). Mechanisms underlying hypothalamic temperature changes during sleep in mammals. *Brain Res.*, 632: 136–142.

Azzaroni, A. and Parmeggiani, P.L. (1995a). Postural and sympathetic influences on brain cooling during the ultradian wake–sleep cycle. *Brain Res.*, 671: 78–82.

Azzaroni, A. and Parmeggiani, P.L. (1995b). Synchronized sleep duration is related to tonic vasoconstriction of thermoregulatory heat exchangers. *J. Sleep Res.*, 4: 41–47.

Baccelli, G., Albertini, R., Mancia, G., *et al.* (1974). Central and reflex regulation of sympathetic vasoconstrictor activity of limb muscle during desynchronized sleep in the cat. *Circ. Res.*, 35: 625–635.

Baccelli, G., Albertini, R., Mancia, G., *et al.* (1978). Control of regional circulation by the sino-aortic reflexes during desynchronized sleep in the cat. *Cardiovasc. Res.*, 12: 523–528.

Baker, M.A. and Hayward, J.N. (1967a). Carotid rete and brain temperature of cats. *Nature*, 216: 139–141.

Baker, M.A. and Hayward, J.N. (1967b). Autonomic basis for the rise in brain temperature during paradoxical sleep. *Science*, 157: 1586–1588.

Barbato, G. and Wehr, T.A. (1998). Homeostatic regulation of REM sleep in humans during extended sleep. *Sleep*, 21: 267–276.

Bard, P., Woods, W.J. and Bleier, R. (1970). The effects of cooling, heating and pyrogen on chronically decerebrated cats. In: Hardy, J.D. *et al.* (eds), *Physiological and Behavioral Temperature Regulation*. Springfield, Ill.:Thomas, 519–543.

Baust, W. and Bohnert, B. (1969). The regulation of hearth rate during sleep. *Exp. Brain Res.*, 7: 169–180.

Behbehani, M.M. and Da Costa, G. (1996). Properties of a projection pathway from the medial preoptic nucleus to the midbrain periaqueductal gray of the rat and its role in the regulation of cardiovascular function. *Brain Res.*, 740: 141–150.

Bellville, J.W., Howland, W.S., Seed, J.C., *et al.* (1959). The effect of sleep on the respiratory response to carbon dioxide. *Anesthesiology*, 20: 628–634.

Benington, J.H. and Heller, H.C. (1994). REM sleep timing is controlled homeostatically by accumulation of REM-sleep propensity in non-REM sleep. *Am. J. Physiol.*, 266: R1992–R2000.

Berger, H. (1929). Ueber das Elektroenkephalogramm des Menschen. *Arch. Psychiatr. Nervenkr.*, 87: 527–570.

Bernard, C. (1865). *Introduction à l'étude de la médicine expérimentale*. Paris: J.B. Baillière.

Bernard, C. (1878–1879). *Leçons sur les phénomènes de la vie communs aux animaux et aux végétaux*. Paris: Museum, vol. I–II.

Berteotti, C., Franzini, C., Lenzi, P., *et al.* (2008). Surges of arterial pressure during rapid-eye-movement sleep in spontaneously hypertensive rats. *Sleep*, 31: 111–117.

Berthon-Jones, M. and Sullivan, C.E. (1982). Ventilatory and arousal responses to hypoxia in sleeping humans. *Am. Rev. Respir. Dis.*, 125: 632–639.

Berthon-Jones, M. and Sullivan, C.E. (1984). Ventilation and arousal responses to hypercapnia in normal sleeping adults. *J. Appl. Physiol.*, 57: 59–67.

Birchfield, R.I., Sieker, H.O. and Heyman, A. (1958). Alterations in blood gases during natural sleep and narcolepsy. *Neurology*, 8: 107–112.

Birchfield, R.I., Sieker, H.O. and Heyman, A. (1959). Alterations in respiratory function during natural sleep. *J. Lab. Clin. Med.*, 54: 216–222.

Bolton, D.P.G. and Herman, S. (1974). Ventilation and sleep state in the newborn. *J. Physiol.*, 240: 67–77.

Borbely, A.A. and Achermann, P. (2005). Sleep homeostasis and models of sleep regulation. In: Kryger, M.H., Roth, T. and Dement, W.C. (eds). *Principles and Practice of Sleep Medicine*. Philadelphia: Elsevier Saunders, 405–417.

Bowes, G., Townsend, E.R., Kozar, L.F., *et al.* (1981). Effect of carotid body denervation on arousal response to hypoxia in sleeping dogs. *J. Appl. Physiol.*, 51: 40–45.

Brazier, M.A.B. (1960). *The electrical activity of the nervous system*. London: Pitman Medical Publishing Co.

Brebbia, D.R. and Altshuler, K.Z. (1965). Oxygen consumption rate and electroencephalographic stage of sleep. *Science*, 150: 1621–1623.

Bremer, F. (1935). Cerveau "isolé" et physiologie du sommeil. *C. R. Soc. Biol.*, 118: 1235–1241.

Bristow, J.D., Honour, A.J., Pickering, T.G., *et al.* (1969). Cardiovascular and respiratory changes during sleep in normal and hypertensive subjects. *Cardiovasc. Res.*, 3: 476–485.

Brown, R.E. and McCarley, R.W. (2005). Neurotransmitters, neuromodulators and sleep. In: Parmeggiani, P.L. and Velluti, R. (eds). *The Physiologic Nature of Sleep*. London: Imperial College Press, 45–75.

Bryan, H.M., Hagan, R., Gulston, G., *et al.* (1976). CO_2 response and sleep state in infants. *Clin. Res.*, 24: A689.

Bülow, K. (1963). Respiration and wakefulness in man. *Acta Physiol. Scand.*, 59: suppl. 209.

Bülow, K. and Ingvar, D.H. (1961). Respiration and state of wakefulness in normals, studied by spirography, capnography and EEG. *Acta Physiol. Scand.*, 51: 230–238.

Busija, D.W. and Heistad, D.D. (1984). Factors involved in the physiological regulation of the cerebral circulation. *Rev. Physiol. Biochem. Pharmacol.*, 101: 162–211.

Calasso, M. and Parmeggiani, P.L. (2004). Thermogenesis of interscapular brown adipose tissue selectively influences pontine and preoptic-hypothalamic temperatures during sleep in the rat. *Brain Res.*, 1015: 103–106.

Calasso, M. and Parmeggiani, P.L. (2008). Carotid blood flow during REM sleep. *Sleep*, 31: 701–707.

Calasso, M., Zantedeschi, E. and Parmeggiani, P.L. (1993). Cold-defense function of brown adipose tissue during sleep. *Am. J. Physiol.*, 265: R1060–R1064.

Campen, M.J., Tagaito, Y., Jenkins, T.P., *et al.* (2002). Phenotipic differences in the hemodynamic response during REM sleep in six strains of inbred mice. *Physiol. Genomics*, 11: 227–234.

Cannon, W.B. (1926). Physiological regulation of normal states: Some tentative postulates concerning biological homeostatics. In: Petitt, A. (ed.). A Charles Richet: Ses Amis, ses Collegues, ses Eleves. Paris: Les Editions Medicales, 91–93.

Cannon, W.B. (1929). Organization for physiological homeostasis. *Physiol. Rev.*, 9: 399–431.

Cannon, W.B. (1932). *The Wisdom of the Body*. New York: Norton.

Capitani, P., Cerri, M., Amici, R., *et al.* (2005). Changes in EEG activity and hypothalamic temperature as indices for non-REM sleep to REM sleep transitions. *Neuroscience Letters*, 383: 182–187.

Caputa, M., Kadziela, W. and Narebski, J. (1976). Significance of cranial circulation for the brain homeothermia in rabbits. II. The role of the cranial venous lakes in the defence against hyperthermia. *Acta Neurobiol. Exp.*, 36: 625–638.

Carrington, M.J., Barbieri, R., Colrain, I.M., *et al.* (2005). Changes in cardiovascular function during the sleep onset period in young adults. *J. Appl. Physiol.*, 98: 468–476.

Caton, R. (1875). The electric currents of the brain. *Brit. Med. J.*, 2: 278.

Cerri, M., Ocampo-Garces, A., Amici, R., *et al.* (2005). Cold exposure and sleep in the rat: effects on sleep architecture and the electroencephalogram. *Sleep*, 28: 694–705.

Cevolani, D. and Parmeggiani, P.L. (1995). Responses of extrahypothalamic neurons to short temperature transients during the ultradian wake–sleep cycle. *Brain Res. Bull.*, 37: 227–232.

Chase, M.H. and Morales, F.R. (2005). Control of motoneurons during sleep. In: Kryger, M.H., Roth, T. and Dement, W.C. (eds). *Principles and Practice of Sleep Medicine*. Philadelphia: Elsevier Saunders, 154–168.

Cianci, T., Zoccoli, G., Lenzi, P., *et al.* (1991). Loss of integrative control of peripheral circulation during desynchronised sleep. *Am. J. Physiol.*, 261: R373–R377.

Cipolli, C. (2005). Sleep and memory. In: Parmeggiani, P.L. and Velluti, R. (eds). *The Physiologic Nature of Sleep*. London: Imperial College Press, 601–629.

Claparède, E. (1905). Esquisse d'une théorie biologique du sommeil. *Arch. Psychol.*, 4: 246–349.

Coccagna, G., Mantovani, M. and Lugaresi, E. (1971). Arterial pressure changes during spontaneous sleep in man. *Electroencephalograph. clin. Neurophysiol.*, 31: 277–281.

Combs, C., Smith, O., Astley, C., *et al.* (1986). Differential effect of behavior on cardiac and vasomotor baroreflex responses. *Am. J. Physiol.*, 251: R126–R136.

Conway, J., Boon, N., Jones, J.V., *et al.* (1983). Involvement of the baroreceptor reflexes in the changes in blood pressure with sleep and mental arousal. *Hypertension*, 5: 746–748.

Cowley, A.W. Jr., Hinojosa-Laborde, C. and Barber, B.J. (1989). Short-term autoregulation of systemic blood flow and cardiac output. *News Physiol. Sci.*, 4: 219–225.

Craig, W. (1918). Appetites and aversion as constituents of instincts. *Biol. Bull.*, 34: 91–107.

Dawes, G.S., Fox, H.E., Leduc, B.M., *et al.* (1972). Respiratory movements and rapid eye movement sleep in the foetal lamb. *J. Physiol.*, 220: 119–143.

Del Bo, A., Baccelli, G., Cellina, G., *et al.* (1985). Carotid sinus reflexes during postural changes, naturally elicited fighting behavior and phases of sleep in the cat. *Cardiovasc. Res.*, 19: 762–769.

Delgado, J.M.R. and Hanai, T. (1966). Intracerebral temperatures in free-moving cats. *Am. J. Physiol.*, 211: 755–769.

Denoyer, M., Sallanon, M., Buda, C., *et al.* (1992). The posterior hypothalamus is responsible for the increase of brain temperature during paradoxical sleep. *Exp. Brain Res.*, 84: 326–334.

Dentico, D., Amici, R. Baracchi, F., *et al.* (2009). c-Fos expression in preoptic nuclei as a marker of sleep rebound in the rat. *Eur. J. Neurosci.*, 30: 651–661.

Dewasmes, G., Bothorel, B., Candas, V., *et al.* (1997). A short-term poikilothermic period occurs just after paradoxical sleep onset in humans: characterization changes in sweating effector activity. *J. Sleep Res.*, 6: 252–258.

Douglas, N.J., White, D.P., Weil, J.V., *et al.* (1982). Hypoxic ventilatory response decreases during sleep in normal men. *Am. Rev. Respir. Dis.*, 125: 286–289.

Dufour, R. and Court, L. (1977). Le débit cérébral sanguin au cours du sommeil paradoxal du lapin. *Arch. Ital. Biol.*, 115: 57–76.

Duron, B. (1969). Activité électrique spontanée des muscles intercostaux et de diaphragme chez l'animal chronique. *J. Physiol.*, 61, suppl 2: 282–283.

Duron, B. (1972). La fonction respiratoire pendant le sommeil physiologique. *Bull. Physio-Path. Resp.*, 8: 1031–1057.

Edvinsson, L., MacKenzie, E.T. and McCulloch, J. (1993). *Cerebral Blood Flow and Metabolism.* New York: Raven Press.

Fagenholz, S.A., O'Connell, K. and Shannon, D.C. (1976). Chemoreceptor function and sleep state in apnea. *Pediatrics*, 58: 31–36.

Farber, J.P. and Marlow, T.A. (1976). Pulmonary reflexes and breathing pattern during sleep in the opossum. *Respir. Physiol.*, 27: 73–86.

Fewell, J.E. (1993). Influence of sleep on systemic and coronary hemodynamics in lambs. *J. Dev. Physiol.*, 19: 71–76.

Feyerabend, P. (1975). *Against Method.* London: Verso.

Finer, N.N., Abroms, I.F. and Taeusch, H.W. Jr. (1976). Ventilation and sleep state in the new born infants. *J. Pediatr.*, 89: 100–108.

Fink, B.R. (1961). Influence of cerebral activity in wakefulness on regulation of breathing. *J. Appl. Physiol.*, 16: 15–20.

Florant, G.L., Turner, B.M. and Heller, H.C. (1978). Temperature regulation during wakefulness, sleep and hibernation in marmots. *Am. J. Physiol.*, 235: R82–R88.

Fort, P., Bassetti, C.L. and Luppi, P.H. (2009). Alternating vigilance states: new insights regarding neuronal networks and mechanisms. *Eur. J. Neurosci.*, 29: 1741–1753.

Frantz, I.D., Adler, S.M., Abroms, I.F., *et al.* (1976). Respiratory responses to airway occlusion in infants: sleep state and maturation. *J. Appl. Physiol.*, 41: 634–638.

Franzini, C. (1992). Brain metabolism and blood flow during sleep. *J. Sleep. Res.*, 1: 3–16.

Franzini, C. (2005). Cardiovascular physiology: the peripheral circulation. In: Kryger, M.H., Roth, T. and Dement, W.C. (eds). *Principles and Practice of Sleep Medicine.* Philadelphia: Elsevier Saunders, 203–212.

Franzini, C., Cianci, T., Lenzi, P., *et al.* (1982). Neural control of vasomotion in rabbit ear is impaired during desynchronized sleep. *Am. J. Physiol.*, 243: R142–R146.

Frysinger, R.C., Marks, J.D., Trelease, R.B., *et al.* (1984). Sleep states attenuate the pressor response to central amygdala stimulation. *Exp. Neurol.*, 83: 604–617.

Gassel, M.M., Ghelarducci, B., Marchiafava, P.L., *et al.* (1964). Phasic changes in blood pressure and heart rate during the rapid eye movement episodes of desynchronized sleep in unrestrained cats. *Arch. Ital. Biol.*, 102: 530–544.

Gebber, G.L., Barman, S.M. and Kocsis, B. (1990). Coherence of medullary unit activity and sympathetic nerve discharge. *Am. J. Physiol.*, 259: R561–R571.

Gillam, P.M.S. (1972). Patterns of respiration in human beings at rest and during sleep. *Bull. Physiopathol. Resp. (Nancy)*, 8: 1059–1070.

Gilmore, J.P. and Tomomatsu, E. (1984). Comparison of carotid sinus baroreceptors in dogs, cats, monkeys and rabbits. *Am. J. Physiol.*, 247: R52–R56.

Glotzbach, S.F. and Heller, H.C. (1976). Central nervous regulation of body temperature during sleep. *Science*, 194: 537–539.

Glotzbach, S.F. and Heller, H.C. (1984). Changes in the thermal characteristics of hypothalamic neurons during sleep and wakefulness. *Brain Res.*, 309: 17–26.

Guazzi, M. and Freis, E.D. (1969). Sinoaortic reflexes and arterial pH, pO_2 and pCO_2 in wakefulness and sleep. *Am. J. Physiol.*, 217: 1623–1627.

Guazzi, M. and Zanchetti, A. (1965). Blood pressure and heart rate during natural sleep of the cat and their regulation by carotid sinus and aortic reflexes. *Arch. Ital. Biol.*, 103: 789–817.

Guazzi, M., Baccelli, G. and Zanchetti, A. (1968). Reflex chemoceptive regulation of arterial pressure during natural sleep in the cat. *Am. J. Phsysiol.*, 214: 969–978.

Hale, A.R. (1960). Circle of Willis: functional concepts, old and new. *Am. Heart. J.*, 60: 491–494.

Haskell, E.H., Palca, J.W., Walker, J.M., *et al.* (1981). Metabolism and thermoregulation during stages of sleep in humans exposed to heat and cold. *J. Appl. Physiol.*, 51: 948–954.

Hathorn, M.K.S. (1974). The rate and depth of breathing in new-born infants in different sleep states. *J. Physiol.*, 243: 101–113.

Hayward, J.N. (1968). Brain temperature regulation during sleep and arousal in the dog. *Exp. Neurol.*, 21: 201–212.

Hayward, J.N. and Baker, M. (1968). A Role of the cerebral arterial blood in the regulation of brain temperature in the monkey. *Am. J. Physiol.*, 215: 389–403.

Hayward, J.N. and Baker, M.A. (1969). A comparative study of the role of the cerebral arterial blood in the regulation of brain temperature in five mammals. *Brain Res.*, 16: 417–440.

Hedemark, L.L. and Kronenberg, R.S. (1982). Ventilatory and heart rate responses to hypoxia and hypercapnia during sleep in adults. *J. Appl. Physiol.*, 53: 307–312.

Hediger, H. (1959). Wie Tiere schlafen. *Med. Klin.*, 20: 938–946.

Hediger, H. (1969). Comparative observations on sleep. *Proc. Roy. Soc. Med.*, 62: 153–156.

Henane, R., Buguet, A., Roussel, B., *et al.* (1977). Variations in evaporation and body temperature during sleep in man. *J. Appl. Physiol.,* 42: 50–55.

Henderson-Smart, D.J. and Read, D.J.C. (1978). Depression of intercostal and abdominal muscle activity and vulnerability to asphyxia during active sleep in the newborn. In: Guilleminault, C. and Dement, W.C. (eds). *Sleep Apnea Syndromes.* New York, NY: A.R. Liss, Kroc Foundation Series, 11: 93–117.

Hendricks, J.C. (1982). Absence of shivering in the cat during paradoxical sleep without atonia. *Exp. Neurol.,* 75: 700–710.

Hendricks, J.C., Bowker, R.M. and Morrison, A.R. (1977). Functional characteristics of cats with pontine lesions during sleep and wakefulness and their usefulness for sleep research. In: Koella, W.P. and Levin, C. (eds). (1976). *Sleep.* Basel: Karger, 207–210.

Hendricks, J.C., Morrison, A.R. and Mann, G.L. (1982). Different behaviors during paradoxical sleep without atonia depend on pontine lesion site. *Brain. Res.,* 239: 81–105.

Henke, K.G., Dempsey, J.A., Badr, M.S., *et al.* (1991). Effect of sleep-induced increases in upper airway resistance on respiratory muscle activity. *J. Appl. Physiol.,* 70: 158–168.

Henke, K.G., Badr, M.S., Skatrud, J.B., *et al.* (1992). Load compensation and respiratory muscle function during sleep. *J. Appl. Physiol.,* 72: 1221–1234.

Henley, K. and Morrison, A.R. (1974). A re-evaluation of the effects of lesions of the pontine tegmentum and locus coeruleus on phenomena of paradoxical sleep in the cat. *Acta Neurobiol. Exp.,* 34: 215–232.

Hensel, H., Brück, K. and Raths, P. (1973). Homeothermic Organisms. In: Precht, H., Christophersen, J., Hensel, H., *et al.* (eds). *Temperature and Life.* Berlin: Springer-Verlag, 503–761.

Hess, W.R. (1944). Das Schlafsyndrom als Folge diencephaler Reizung. *Helv. Physiol. Acta,* 2: 305–344.

Hinde, R.A. (1966). *Animal Behavior.* New York: McGraw-Hill.

Hirasawa, M., Nishihara, M. and Takahashi, M. (1996). The rostral ventrolateral medulla mediates suppression of the circulatory system by the ventromedial nucleus of the hypothalamus. *Brain Res.,* 724: 186–190.

Holzapfel, M. (1940). Triebbedingte Ruhezustände als Ziel von Appetenzhandlungen. *Naturwissenshaften,* 28: 273–280.

Horne, R.S.C., De Preu, N.D., Berger, P.J., *et al.* (1991). Arousal responses to hypertension in lambs: Effect of sinoaortic denervation. *Am. J. Physiol.,* 260: H1283–H1289.

Hosoya, Y., Sugiura, Y., Okado, N., *et al.* (1991). Descending input from the hypothalamic paraventricular nucleus to sympathetic preganglionic neurons in the rat. *Exp. Brain Res.,* 85: 10–20.

Huber, R., Hill, S.L., Holladay, C., *et al.* (2004). Sleep homeostasis in *Drosophila Melanogaster. Sleep,* 27: 628–639.

Iellamo, F., Placidi, F., Marciani, M.G., *et al.* (2004). Baroreflex buffering of sympathetic activation during sleep: evidence from autonomic assessment of sleep macroarchitecture and microarchitecture. *Hypertension,* 43: 814–819.

Islas-Marroquin, J. (1966). L'activité des muscles respiratoires pendant les différentes phases du sommeil physiologiques chez le chat. *Arch. Sci. Physiol.*, 20: 219–231.

I.U.P.S. Commission for Thermal Physiology. (1987). Glossary of Terms for Thermal Physiology. *Pflugers Arch.*, 410: 567–587.

Iwamura, Y., Uchino, Y., Ozawa, S., *et al.* (1969). Spontaneous and reflex discharge of a sympathetic nerve during "para-sleep" in decerebrate cat. *Brain Res.*, 16: 359–367.

Jones, J.V., Sleight, P. and Smyth, H.S. (1982). Haemodynamic changes during sleep in man. In: Ganten, D. and Pfaff, D. (eds). *Sleep. Current Topics in Endocrinology*. New York, NY: Academic Press, 213–272.

Jouvet, M. (1962). Recherches sur le structures nerveuses et les mechanismes responsables des differentes phases du sommeil physiologique. *Arch. Ital. Biol.*, 100: 125–206.

Jouvet, M. and Delorme, F. (1965). Locus coeruleus et sommeil paradoxal. *C. R. Soc. Biol.*, 159: 895–899.

Junqueira, L.F. Jr. and Krieger, E.M. (1976). Blood pressure and sleep in the rat in normotension and in neurogenic hypertension. *J. Physiol.*, 259: 725–735.

Kanosue, K., Yanase-Fujiwara, M. and Hosono, T. (1994a). Hypothalamic network for thermoregulatory vasomotor control. *Am. J. Physiol.*, 267: R283–R288.

Kanosue, K., Zhang, Y.H., Yanase-Fujiwara, M., *et al.* (1994b). Hypothalamic network for thermoregulatory shivering. *Am. J. Physiol.*, 267: R275–R282.

Kanzow, E., Krause, D. and Kühnel, H. (1962). Die Vasomotorik der Hirnrinde in den Phasen desynchronisierter EEG Aktivität im natürlichen Schlaf der Katze. *Pflügers Arch. Gesamte Physiol.*, 274: 593–607.

Kawamura, H. and Sawyer, C.H. (1965). Elevation in brain temperature during paradoxical sleep. *Science*, 150: 912–913.

Kawamura, H., Withmoyer, D.I. and Sawyer, C.H. (1966). Temperature changes in the rabbit brain during paradoxical sleep. *Electroencephalogr. Clin. Neurophysiol.*, 21: 469–477.

Khatri, I.M. and Freis, E.D. (1967). Hemodynamic changes during sleep. *J. Appl. Physiol.*, 22: 867–873.

Kleitman, N. (1963). *Sleep and Wakefulness*. Chicago: The University of Chicago Press.

Knill, R., Andrews, W., Bryan, A.C., *et al.* (1976). Respiratory load compensation in infants. *J. Appl. Physiol.*, 40: 357–361.

Knuepfer, M.M., Stumpf, H. and Stock, G. (1986). Baroreceptor sensitivity during desynchronized sleep. *Exp. Neurol.*, 92: 323–334.

Kräuchi, K., Cajochen, C. and Wirz-Justice, A. (1997). A relationship between heat loss and sleepiness: effects of postural change and melatonin administration. *J. Appl. Physiol.*, 83: 134–139.

Kräuchi, K., Cajochen, C., Werth, E., *et al.* (1999). Warm feet promotes the rapid onset of sleep. *Nature*, 401: 36–37.

Kräuchi, K., Cajochen, C., Werth, E., *et al.* (2000). Functional link between distal vasodilation and sleep-onset latency. *Am. J. Physiol.*, 278: R741–R748.

Kryger, M.H., Roth, T. and Dement, W.C. (eds). *Principles and Practice of Sleep Medicine*. Philadelphia: Elsevier Saunders, 2005.

Kumazawa, T., Baccelli, G., Guazzi, M., *et al.* (1969). Hemodynamic patterns during desynchronized sleep in intact cats and in cats with sinoaortic deafferentation. *Circ. Res.*, 24: 923–937.

Lacombe, J., Nosjean, A., Meunier, J.M., *et al.* (1988). Computer analysis of cardiovascular changes during sleep–wake cycle in Sprague–Dawley rats. *Am. J. Physiol.*, 254: H217–H222.

Lashley, K.S. (1938). Experimental analysis of instinctive behaviour. *Psychol. Rev.*, 45: 445–471.

Lenzi, P., Cianci, T., Guidalotti, P.L., *et al.* (1987). Brain circulation during sleep and its relation to extracerebral hemodynamics. *Brain Res.*, 415: 14–20.

Libert, J.P. and Bach, V. (2005). Thermoregulation and sleep in the human. In: Parmeggiani, P.L. and Velluti, R. (eds). *The Physiologic Nature of Sleep*. London: Imperial College Press, 407–431.

Lorenz, K. (1956). The objectivistic theory of instinct. In: Grasse, P.P. (ed.). *L'Instinct dans le Comportement des Animaux et de l'Homme*. Paris: Masson, 51–76.

Lu, J., Sherman, D., Devor, M., *et al.* (2006). A putative flip-flop switch for control of REM sleep. *Nature*, 441: 589–594.

Lugaresi, E., Coccagna, G., Mantovani, M., *et al.* (1972). Some periodic phenomena arising during drowsiness and sleep in man. *Electroencephalogr. Clin. Neurophysiol.*, 32: 701–705.

Luppi, M., Martelli, D., Amici, R., *et al.* (2010). Hypothalamic osmoregulation is maintained across the wake–sleep cycle in the rat. *J. Sleep Res.*, 19: 394–399.

Lydic, R. and Orem, J. (1979). Respiratory neurons of the pneumotaxic center during sleep and wakefulness. *Neuroscience Letters*, 15: 187–192.

Mancia, G. (1993). Autonomic modulation of the cardiovascular system during sleep. *N. Engl. J. Med.*, 328: 347–349.

Mancia, G. and Zanchetti, A. (1980). Cardiovascular regulation during sleep. In: Orem, J. and Barnes, C.D. (eds). *Physiology in Sleep. Research Topics in Physiology*. New York, NY: Academic Press, vol. 3: 1–55.

Mancia, G., Baccelli, G., Adams, D.B., *et al.* (1971). A vasomotor regulation during sleep in the cat. *Am. J. Physiol.*, 83: 1086–1093.

Maquet, P. (2000). Functional neuroimaging of normal human sleep by positron emission tomography. *J. Sleep Res.*, 9: 207–231.

Marks, J.D., Frysinger, R.C. and Harper, R.M. (1987). State-dependent respiratory depression elicited by stimulation of the orbital frontal cortex. *Exp. Neurol.*, 95: 714–729.

McGinty, D., Alam, M.N., Szymusiak, R., *et al.* (2001). Hypothalamic sleep-promoting mechanisms: coupling to thermoregulation. *Arch. Ital. Biol.*, 139: 63–75.

McGinty, D., Alam, N., Suntsova, N., *et al.* (2005). Hypothalamic mechanisms of sleep: perspective from neuronal unit recording studies. In: Parmeggiani, P.L. and Velluti, R. (eds). *The Physiologic Nature of Sleep*. London: Imperial College Press, 139–160.

Meunier, J.M., Nosjean, A., Lacombe, J., *et al.* (1988). Cardiovascular changes during the sleep-wake cycle in spontaneous hypertensive rats and in their genetically normotensive precursors. *Pflügers Arch.*, 411: 195–199.

Miki, K., Kato, M. and Kajii, S. (2003). Relationship beween renal sympathetic nerve activity and arterial pressure during REM sleep in rats. *Am. J. Physiol.*, 284: R467–R473.

Miki, K., Oda, M., Kamijyo, N., *et al.* (2004). Lumbar sympathetic nerve activity and hindquarter blood flow during REM sleep in rats. *J. Physiol.*, 557: 261–271.

Mitchell, R.A. and Berger, A.J. (1975). Neural regulation of respiration. *Am. Rev. Respir. Dis.*, 111: 206–224.

Monti, A., Medigue, C., Nedelcoux, H., *et al.* (2002). Autonomic control of the cardiovascular system during sleep in normal subjects. *Eur. J. Appl. Physiol.*, 87: 174–181.

Moore-Ede, M.C. (1986). Physiology of the circadian timing system: Predictive versus reactive homeostasis. *Am. J. Physiol.*, 250: R737–R752.

Morrison, A.R. (2005). The power of behavioral analysis in understanding sleep mechanisms. In: Parmeggiani, P.L. and Velluti, R. (eds). *The Physiologic Nature of Sleep*. London: Imperial College Press, 187–206.

Moruzzi, G. (1969). Sleep and instinctive behavior. *Arch. Ital. Biol.*, 107: 175–216.

Moruzzi, G. and Magoun, H.W. (1949). Brain stem reticular formation and activation of the EEG. *Electroencephalogr. Clin. Neurophysiol.*, 1: 455–473.

Mrosovsky, N. (1990). *Rheostasis.The Physiology of Change*. New York: Oxford University Press.

Mukhametov, L.M., Lyamin, O.I. and Polyakova, I.G. (1985). Interhemispheric asynchrony of the sleep EEG in northern fur seals. *Experientia*, 41: 1034–1035.

Nagura, S., Sakagami, T., Kakiichi, A., *et al.* (2004). Acute shifts in baroreflex control of renal sympathetic nerve activity induced by REM sleep and grooming in rats. *J. Physiol.*, 558: 975–983.

Nakazato, T., Shikama, T., Toma, S., *et al.* (1998). Nocturnal variation in human sympathetic baroreflex sensitivity. *J. Auton. Nerv. Syst.*, 70: 32–37.

Netick, A. and Foutz, A.S. (1980). Respiratory activity and sleep–wakefulness in the deafferented paralised cat. *Sleep*, 3: 1–12.

Netick, A., Dugger, W.J. and Symmons, R.A. (1984). Ventilatory response to hypercapnia during sleep and wakefulness in cats. *J. Appl. Physiol.*, 56: 1347–1354.

Ninomiya, I., Akiyama, T. and Nishiura, N. (1990). Mechanism of cardiac-related synchronized cardiac sympathetic nerve activity in awake cats. *Am. J. Physiol.*, 259: R499–R506.

Noble, D. and Boyd, C.A.R. (1993). The challenge of integrative physiology. In: Noble, D. and Boyd, C.A.R. (eds). *The Logic of Life*. Oxford: Oxford University Press, 1–13.

Noll, G., Elam, M. and Kunimoto, M. (1994). Skin sympathetic nerve activity and effector function during sleep in humans. *Acta Physiol. Scand.*, 151: 319–329.

Obal, F. Jr., Tobler, I. and Borbely, A. (1983). Effect of ambient temperature on the 24-hour sleep–wake cycle in normal and capsaicin-treated rats. *Physiol. Behav.*, 30: 425–430.

Orem, J. (1980). Neuronal mechanisms of respiration in REM sleep. *Sleep*, 3: 251–267.

Orem, J., Montplaisir, J. and Dement, W.C. (1974). Changes in the activity of respiratory neurons during sleep. *Brain Res.*, 82: 309–315.

Orem, J., Netick, A. and Dement, W.C. (1977a). Increased upper airway resistance to breathing during sleep in the cat. *Electroencephalogr. Clin. Neurophysiol.*, 43: 14–22.

Orem, J., Netick, A. and Dement, W.C. (1977b). Breathing during sleep and wakefulness in the cat. *Respir. Physiol.*, 30: 265–289.

Palca, J.W., Walker, J.M. and Berger, R.J. (1986). Thermoregulation, metabolism and stages of sleep in cold-exposed men. *J. Appl. Physiol.*, 61: 940–947.

Parmeggiani, P.L. (1960). Reizeffekte aus Hippocampus und Corpus mammillare der Katze. *Helv. Physiol. Acta*, 18: 523–536.

Parmeggiani, P.L. (1962). Sleep behaviour elicited by electrical stimulation of cortical and subcortical structures in the cat. *Helv. Physiol. Acta*, 20: 347–367.

Parmeggiani, P.L. (1968). Telencephalo-diencephalic aspects of sleep mechanisms. *Brain Res.*, 7: 350–359.

Parmeggiani, P.L. (1973). The physiological role of sleep. In: Levin, P. and Koella, W.P. (eds). *Sleep*. Basel: Karger, 210–216.

Parmeggiani, P.L. (1978). Regulation of the activity of respiratory muscles during sleep. In: Fitzgerald, R.S., Gautier, H. and Lahiri, S. (eds). *Advances in Experimental Medicine and Biology*. New York, NY: Plenum Press, 47–57.

Parmeggiani, P.L. (1979). Integrative aspects of hypothalamic influences on respiratory brain-stem mechanisms during wakefulness and sleep. In: von Euler, C. and Lagerkrantz, H. (eds). *Central Nervous Control Mechanisms in Breathing*. Oxford: Pergamon Press, 53–68.

Parmeggiani, P.L. (1980a). Behavioral phenomenology of sleep (somatic and vegetative). *Experientia*, 36: 6–11.

Parmeggiani, P.L. (1980b). Temperature regulation during sleep: A study in homeostasis. In Orem, J. and Barnes, C.D. (eds): *Physiology in Sleep. Research Topics in Physiology*. New York: Academic Press, vol 3: 97–143.

Parmeggiani, P.L. (1982). Regulation of physiological functions during sleep in mammals. *Experientia*, 38: 1405–1408.

Parmeggiani, P.L. (1985). Homeostatic regulation during sleep: Facts and hypotheses. In: McGinty, D.J., Drucker-Colin, R., Morrison, A.R., *et al.* (eds). *Brain Mechanisms of Sleep*. New York: Raven Press, 385–397.

Parmeggiani, P.L. (1987). Interaction between sleep and thermoregulation: An aspect of the control of behavioral states. *Sleep*, 10: 426–435.

Parmeggiani, P.L. (1991). Physiological risks during sleep. In: Peter, J.H., Penzel, T., Podszus, T., *et al.* (eds). *Sleep and Health Risk*. Berlin: Springer-Verlag, 119–123.

Parmeggiani, P.L. (1994). The autonomic nervous system in sleep. In: Kryger, M.H., Roth, T. and Dement, W.C. (eds). *Principles and Practice of Sleep Medicine*. Philadelphia: Saunders, 194–203.

Parmeggiani, P.L. (2005a). The problem of causal determination of sleep behaviour. In: Parmeggiani, P.L. and Velluti, R.A. (eds). *The Physiologic Nature of Sleep*. London: Imperial College Press, 267–278.

Parmeggiani, P.L. (2005b). Sleep behaviour and temperature. In: Parmeggiani, P.L. and Velluti, R.A. (eds). *The Physiologic Nature of Sleep*. London: Imperial College Press, 387–405.

Parmeggiani, P.L. and Rabini, C. (1967). Shivering and panting during sleep. *Brain Res.*, 6: 789–791.

Parmeggiani, P.L. and Rabini, C. (1970). Sleep and environmental temperature. *Arch. Ital. Biol.*, 108: 369–387.

Parmeggiani, P.L. and Sabattini, L. (1972): Electromyographic aspects of postural, respiratory and thermoregulatory mechanisms in sleeping cats. *Electroencephalogr. Clin. Neurophysiol.*, 33: 1–13.

Parmeggiani, P.L., Rabini, C. and Cattalani, M. (1969). Sleep phases at low environmental temperature. *Arch. Sci. Biol.*, 53: 277–290.

Parmeggiani, P.L., Franzini, C., Lenzi, P., *et al.* (1971). Inguinal subcutaneous temperature changes in cats sleeping at different environmental temperatures. *Brain Res.*, 33: 397–404.

Parmeggiani, P.L., Franzini, C., Lenzi, P., *et al.* (1973). Threshold of respiratory responses to preoptic heating during sleep in freely moving cats. *Brain Res.*, 52: 189–201.

Parmeggiani, P.L., Zamboni, G., Cianci, T., *et al.* (1974). Influence of anterior hypothalamic heating on the duration of fast-wave sleep episodes. *Electroencephalogr. Clin. Neurophysiol.*, 36: 465–470.

Parmeggiani, P.L., Agnati, L.F., Zamboni, G., *et al.* (1975). Hypothalamic temperature during the sleep cycle at different ambient temperatures. *Electroencephalogr. Clin. Neurophysiol.*, 38: 589–596.

Parmeggiani, P.L., Franzini, C. and Lenzi, P. (1976). Respiratory frequency as a function of preoptic temperature during sleep. *Brain Res.*, 111: 253–260.

Parmeggiani, P.L., Zamboni, G., Cianci, T., *et al.* (1977). Absence of thermoregulatory vasomotor responses during fast wave sleep in cats. *Electroenceph. Clin. Neurophysiol.*, 42: 372–380.

Parmeggiani, P.L., Cianci, T., Calasso, M., *et al.* (1980). Quantitative analysis of short term deprivation and recovery of desynchronized sleep in cats. *Electroencephalogr. Clin. Neurophysiol.*, 50: 293–302.

Parmeggiani, P.L., Calasso, M. and Cianci, T. (1981). Respiratory effects of preoptic-anterior hypothalamic electrical stimulation during sleep in cats. *Sleep*, 4: 71–82.

Parmeggiani, P.L., Azzaroni, A., Cevolani, D., *et al.* (1983). Responses of anterior hypothalamic-preoptic neurons to direct thermal stimulation during wakefulness and sleep. *Brain Res.*, 269: 382–385.

Parmeggiani, P.L., Zamboni, G., Perez, E., *et al.* (1984). Hypothalamic temperature during desynchronized sleep. *Exp. Brain Res.*, 54: 315–320.

Parmeggiani, P.L., Azzaroni, A., Cevolani, D., *et al.* (1986). Polygraphic study of anterior hypothalamic-preoptic neuron thermosensitivity during sleep. *Electroencephalogr. Clin. Neurophysiol.*, 63: 289–295.

Parmeggiani, P.L., Cevolani, D., Azzaroni, A., *et al.* (1987). Thermosensitivity of anterior hypothalamic-preoptic neurons during the waking–sleeping cycle: a study in brain functional states. *Brain Res.*, 415: 79–89.

Parmeggiani, P.L., Azzaroni, A. and Calasso, M. (1998). A pontine-hypothalamic temperature difference correlated with cutaneous and respiratory heat loss. *Respir. Physiol.*, 114: 49–56.

Parmeggiani, P.L., Azzaroni, A. and Calasso, M. (2002). Systemic hemodynamic changes raising brain temperature in REM sleep. *Brain Res.*, 940: 55–60.

Peyron, C., Tighe, D.K., van den Pol, A.N., *et al.* (1998). Neurons containing hypocretin (orexin) project to multiple neuronal systems. *J. Neurosci.*, 18: 9996–10015.

Phillipson, E.A. (1977). Regulation of breathing during sleep. *Am. Rev. Respir. Dis.*, 115 (suppl.): 217–224.

Phillipson, E.A. (1978). Respiratory adaptations in sleep. *Ann. Rev. Physiol.*, 40: 133–156.

Phillipson, E.A. and Bowes, G. (1986). Control of breathing during sleep. In: Cherniack, N.S. and Widdicombbe, J.G. (eds). *Handbook of Physiology, Section III. The Respiratory System*. Bethesda, MD: American Physiological Society, 642–689.

Phillipson, E.A., Murphy, E. and Kozar, L.F. (1976a). Regulation of respiration in sleeping dogs. *J. Appl. Physiol.*, 40: 688–693.

Phillipson, E.A., Kozar, L.F. and Murphy, E. (1976b). Respiratory load compensation in awake and sleeping dogs. *J. Appl. Physiol.*, 40: 895–902.

Phillipson, E.A., Kozar, L.F., Rebuck, A.S., *et al.* (1977). Ventilatory and waking responses to CO_2 in sleeping dogs. *Am. Rev. Respir. Dis.*, 115: 251–259.

Phillipson, E.A., Sullivan, C.E., Read, D.J.C., *et al.* (1978). Ventilatory and waking responses to hypoxia in sleeping dogs. *J. Appl. Physiol.*, 44: 512–520.

Prudom, A.E. and Klemm, W.R. (1973). Electrographic correlates of sleep behavior in a primitive mammal, the armadillo *Dasypus novemcinctus*. *Physiol. Behav.*, 10: 275–282.

Puizillout, J.J., Ternaux, J.P., Foutz, A.S., *et al.* (1974). Les stades de sommeil chez la préparation "encéphale isolé". 1. Déclenchement des pointes ponto-géniculo-occipitales et du sommeil phasique à ondes lentes. Role des noyaux du raphé. *Electroencephalogr. Clin. Neurophysiol.*, 37: 561–576.

Purcell, M. (1976). Response in the newborn to raised upper airway resistance. *Arch. Child. Dis.*, 51: 602–607.

Rechtschaffen, A. and Kales, A. (1968). *A Manual of Standardized Terminology, Techniques and Scoring System for Sleep Stages of Human Subjects*. Los Angeles: B.I.S./B.R.I., U.C.L.A.

Reed, D.J. and Kellogg, R.H. (1958). Changes in respiratory response to CO_2 during natural sleep at sea level and at altitude. *J. Appl. Physiol.*, 13: 325–330.

Reed, D.J. and Kellogg, R.H. (1960). Effect of sleep on hypoxic stimulation of breathing at sea level and altitude. *J. Appl. Physiol.*, 15: 1130–1134.

Reite, M., Jackson, D., Cahoon, R.L., *et al.* (1975). Sleep physiology at high altitude. *Electroencephalogr. Clin. Neurophysiol.*, 38: 463–471.

Reivich, M. (1972). Regional cerebral blood flow in physiologic and pathophysiologic states. In: Meyer, J.S. and Schadé, J.P. (eds). *Cerebral Blood Flow. Progress in Brain Research*, vol. 35. Amsterdam: Elsevier, 191–228.

Remmers, J.E., Bartlett, D. Jr. and Putnam, M.D. (1976). Changes in the respiratory cycle associated with sleep. *Respir. Physiol.*, 28: 227–238.

Risberg, J. and Ingvar, D.H. (1973). Increase of regional cerebral blood volume during REM-sleep in man. In: Koella, W.P. and Levin, P. (eds). *Sleep: Proceedings of the First European Congress on Sleep Research*. Basel: Karger, 384–388.

Roberts, W.W. and Robinson, T.C.L. (1969). Relaxation and sleep induced by warming of the preoptic region and anterior hypothalamus in cats. *Exp. Neurol.*, 25: 282–294.

Roberts, W.W., Bergquist, E.H. and Robinson, T.C.L. (1969). Thermoregulatory grooming and sleep-like relaxation induced by local warming of preoptic area and anterior hypothalamus in opossum. *J. Comp. Physiol. Psychol.*, 67: 182–188.

Robin, E.D., Whaley, R.D., Crump, G.H., et al. (1958). Alveolar gas tension, pulmonary ventilation and blood pH during physiological sleep in normal subjects. *J. Clin. Invest.*, 37: 981–989.

Roussel, B. and Bittel, J. (1979). Thermogenesis and thermolysis during sleeping and waking in the rat. *Pfluegers Arch.*, 382: 225–231.

Roussel, B., Dittmar, A. and Chouvet, G. (1980). Internal temperature variations during the sleep wake cycle in the rat. *Waking Sleeping*, 4: 63–75.

Sagot, J.C., Amoros, C., Candas, V., et al. (1987). Sweating responses and body temperatures during nocturnal sleep in humans. *Am. J. Physiol.*, 252: R462–R470.

Sakaguchi, S., Glotzbach, S.F. and Heller, H.C. (1979). Influence of hypothalamic and ambient temperatures on sleep in kangaroo rats. *Am. J. Physiol.*, 294: R80–R88.

Santiago, T.V., Sinha, A.K. and Edelman, N.H. (1981). Respiratory flow-resistive load compensation during sleep. *Am. Rev. Respir. Dis.*, 123: 382–387.

Santiago, T.V., Scardella, A.T. and Edelman, N.H. (1984). Determinants of the ventilatory response to hypoxia during sleep. *Am. Rev. Respir. Dis.*, 130: 179–182.

Saper, C.B., Chou, T.C. and Scammell T.E. (2001). The sleep switch: hypothalamic control of sleep and wakefulness. *Trends in Neurosciences*, 24: 726–731.

Sastre, J.P. and Jouvet, M. (1979). Oneiric behaviour in cats. *Physiol. Behav.*, 22: 979–989.

Satinoff, E. (1978). Neural organization and evolution of thermal regulation in mammals. *Science*, 201: 16–22.

Satoh, T. (1968). Brain temperature of the cat during sleep. *Arch. Ital. Biol.*, 106: 73–82.

Scharf, S.M. (1984). Influence of sleep state and breathing on cardiovascular function. In: Saunders, N.A. and Sullivan, C.E. (eds). *Sleep and Breathing*. New York, NY: Dekker, vol 21, 221–239.

Schaub, C.D., Tankersley, C., Schwartz, A.R., et al. (1998). Effect of sleep/wake state on arterial blood pressure in genetically identical mice. *J. Appl. Physiol.*, 85: 366–371.

Schmidek, W.R., Hoshino, K., Schmidek, M., et al. (1972). Influence of environmental temperature on the sleep wakefulness cycle in the rat. *Physiol. Behav.*, 8: 363–371.

Schneider, H., Schaub, C.D., Andreoni, K.A., et al. (1997). Systemic and pulmonary hemodynamic responses to normal and obstructed breathing during sleep. *J. Appl. Physiol.*, 83: 1671–1680.

Schulkin, J. (2003). *Rethinking Homeostasis: Allotonic Regulation in Physiology and Patophysiology*. Cambridge: The MIT Press.

Sei, H. and Morita, Y. (1996a). Effect of ambient temperature on arterial pressure variability during sleep in the rat. *Physiol. Behav.*, 55: 37–41.

Sei, H. and Morita, Y. (1996b). Acceleration of EEG theta wave precedes the phasic surge of arterial pressure during REM sleep in the rat. *Neuroreport*, 7: 3059–3062.

Sei, H., Morita, Y., Morita, H., *et al.* (1989). Long-term profiles of sleep-related hemody-namic changes in the postoperative chronic cat. *Physiol. Behav.*, 46: 499–502.

Sei, H., Sakai, K., Kanamori, N., *et al.* (1994). Long-term variations of arterial blood pres-sure during sleep in freely moving cats. *Physiol. Behav.*, 55: 673–679.

Sei, H., Morita, Y., Tsunooka, K., *et al.* (1999). Sino-aortic denervation augments the increase in blood pressure seen during paradoxical sleep in the rat. *J. Sleep Res.*, 8: 45–50.

Sei, H., Sano, A., Ohno, H., *et al.* (2002). Age-related changes in control of blood pressure and heart rate during sleep in the rat. *Sleep*, 25: 279–285.

Serota, H.M. (1939). Temperature changes in the cortex and hypothalamus during sleep. *J. Neurophysiol.*, 2: 42–47.

Serota, H.M. and Gerard, R.W. (1938). Localised thermal changes in the cat's brain. *J. Neurophysiol.*, 1: 115–124.

Sewitch, D.E., Kittrell, E.M.W., Kupfer, D.J., *et al.* (1986). Body temperature and sleep architecture in response to a mild cold stress in women. *Physiol. Behav.*, 36: 951–957.

Seylaz, J., Mamo, H., Goas, J.Y., *et al.* (1971). Local cortical blood flow during paradoxical sleep in man. *Arch. Ital .Biol.*, 109: 1–14.

Shapiro, C.M. and Rosendorff, C. (1975). Local hypothalamic blood flow during sleep. *Electroencephalogr. Clin. Neurophysiol.*, 39: 365–369.

Shapiro, C.M., Moore, A.T., Mitchell, D., *et al.* (1974). How well does man thermoregulate during sleep? *Experientia*, 30: 1279–1281.

Sherin, J.E., Elmquist, J.K., Torrealba, F., *et al.* (1998) Innervation of histaminergic tubero-mammillary neurons by GABAergic and galaninergic neurons in the ventrolateral preoptic nucleus of the rat. *J. Neurosci.*, 18: 4705–4721.

Sichieri, R. and Schmidek, W.R. (1984). Influence of ambient temperature on the sleep — wakefulness cycle in the golden hamster. *Physiol. Behav.*, 33: 871–877.

Siegel, J.M. and Rogawski, M.A. (1988). A function of REM sleep: regulation of noradren-ergic receptor sensitivity. *Brain Res. Rev.*, 13: 213–233.

Siegel, J.M. (2005). REM sleep. In: Kryger, M.H., Roth, T. and Dement, W.C. (eds). *Principles and Practice of Sleep Medicine*. Philadelphia: Elsevier Saunders, 120–135.

Silvani, A. (2008). Physiological sleep-dependent changes in arterial blood pressure: central autonomic commands and baroreflex control. *Clin. Exp. Pharmacol. Physiol.*, 35: 987–994.

Silvani, A. and Lenzi, P. (2005). Reflex cardiovascular control in sleep. In: Parmeggiani, P.L. and Velluti, R.A. (eds), *The Physiologic Nature of Sleep*. London: Imperial College Press, 323–349.

Silvani, A., Bojic, T., Cianci, T., *et al.* (2003). Effects of acoustic stimulation on cardiovas-cular regulation during sleep. *Sleep*, 26: 201–205.

Sindrup, J.H., Kastrup, J., Madsen, P.L., *et al.* (1992). Nocturnal variations in human lower leg subcutaneous blood flow related to sleep stages. *J. Appl. Physiol.*, 73: 1246–1252.

Snyder, F., Hobson, J.A., Morrison, D.F., *et al.* (1964). Changes in respiration, heart rate and systolic blood pressure in human sleep. *J. Appl. Physiol.*, 19: 417–422.

Somers, W.K., Dyken, M.E., Mark, A.L., et al. (1993). Sympathetic nerve activity during sleep in normal subjects. N. Engl. J. Med., 328: 303–307.

Specht, H. and Fruhmann, G. (1972). Incidence of periodic breathing in 2000 subjects without pulmonary or neurological disease. Bull. Physio-Pathol. Respir., 8: 1075.

Sterman, M.B. and Clemente, C.D. (1962). Forebrain inhibitory mechanisms: sleep patterns induced by basal forebrain stimulation in the behaving cat. Exp. Neurol., 6: 103–117.

Sullivan, C.E., Murphy, E., Kozar, L.F., et al. (1979). Ventilatory responses to CO_2 and lung inflation in tonic versus phasic REM sleep. J. Appl. Physiol., 47: 1305–1310.

Szymusiak, R. and Satinoff, E. (1981). Maximal REM sleep time defines a narrower thermoneutral zone than does minimal metabolic rate. Physiol. Behav., 26: 687–690.

Szymusiak, R., Steiniger, T., Alam, M.N., et al. (2001). Preoptic area sleep-regulating mechanisms. Arch. It. Biol., 139: 77–92.

Tachibana, S. (1969). Relation between hypothalamic heat production and intra- and extracranial circulatory factors. Brain Res., 16: 405–416.

Tank, J., Diedrich, A., Hale, N., et al. (2003). Relationship between blood pressure, sleep K-complexes and muscle sympathetic nerve activity in humans. Am. J. Physiol., 285: R208–R214.

Thach, B.T., Abroms, I.F., Frantz, I.D., et al. (1977). REM sleep breathing pattern without intercostal muscle influence. Fed. Proc. 36: 445.

Tinbergen, N. (1951). The Study of Instinct. Oxford: Oxford University Press.

Tononi, G. and Cirelli, C. (2005). A possible role for sleep in synaptic homeostasis. In: Parmeggiani, P.L. and Velluti, R. (eds). The Physiologic Nature of Sleep. London: Imperial College Press, 77–101.

Trinder, J., Whitworth, F., Kay, A., et al. (1992). Respiratory instability during sleep onset. J. Appl. Physiol., 73: 2462–2469.

Tusiewicz, K., Moldofsky, H., Bryan, A.C., et al. (1977). Mechanics of the rib cage and diaphragm during sleep. J. Appl. Physiol., 43: 600–602.

Ursin, R. (1970). Sleep stage relation within the sleep cycles in the cat. Brain Res., 11: 91–97.

Valatx, J.L., Bugat, R. and Jouvet, M. (1972). Genetic studies of sleep in mice. Nature, 238: 226–227.

Valatx, J.L., Roussel, B. and Curé, M. (1973). Sommeil et température cérébrale du rat au cours de l'exposition chronique en ambiance chaude. Brain Res., 55: 107–122.

Valatx, J.L. and Bugat, R. (1974). Facteurs génétiques dans le déterminisme du cycle veille-sommeil chez le souris. Brain Res., 69: 315–330.

van de Borne, P., Nguyen, H., Biston, P., et al. (1994). Effects of wake and sleep stages on the 24-h autonomic control of blood pressure and heart rate in recumbent men. Am. J. Physiol., 266: H548–H554.

van Someren, E.J.W. (2000). More than a marker: interaction between the circadian regulation of temperature and sleep, age-related changes and treatment possibilities. Chronobiol. Int., 17: 313–354.

van Twyver, H. and Allison, T. (1974). Sleep in the armadillo Dasypus Novemcinctus at moderate and low ambient temperatures. Brain Behav. Evol., 9: 107–120.

Velluti, R.A. (2008). *The Auditory System in Sleep*. London: Academic Press (Elsevier).

Villablanca, J. (1966). Behavioral and polygraphic study of "sleep" and "wakefulness" in chronic decerebrate cats. *Electroencephalogr. Clin. Neurophysiol.*, 21: 562–577.

Vivaldi, E.A., Ocampo, A., Wyeneken, U., *et al.* (1994). Short-term homeostasis of active sleep and the architecture of sleep in the rat. *J. Neurophysiol.*, 72: 1745–1755.

von Euler, C. (1964). The gain of the hypothalamic temperature regulating mechanisms. In: Bargman, W. and Schadé, J.P. (eds). *Lectures on the Diencephalon*. Amsterdam: Elsevier, 127–131.

von Euler, C. and Söderberg, U. (1957). The influence of hypothalamic thermoceptive structures on the electroencephalogram and gamma motor activity. *Electroencephalogr. Clin. Neurophysiol.*, 42: 112–129.

Walker, J.M., Walker, L.E., Harris, D.V., *et al.* (1983). Cessation of thermoregulation during REM sleep in the pocket mouse. *Am. J. Physiol.*, 244: R114–R118.

Webb, P. and Hiestand, M. (1975). Sleep metabolism and age. *J. Appl. Physiol.*, 38: 257–262.

White, D.P. (1986). Occlusion pressure and ventilation during sleep in normal humans. *J. Appl. Physiol.*, 61: 1279–1287.

Wiegand, L., Zwillich, C.W., Wiegand, D., *et al.* (1991). Changes in upper airway muscle activation and ventilation during phasic REM sleep in normal men. *J. Appl. Physiol.*, 71: 488–497.

Wurtz, R.H. and O'Flaerty, J.J. (1967). Physiological correlates of steady potential shifts during sleep and wakefulness. 1. Sensitivity of the steady potential to alterations in carbon dioxide. *Electroencephalogr. Clin. Neurophysiol.*, 22: 30–42.

Yoshimoto, M., Sakagami, T., Nagura, S., *et al.* (2004). Relationship between renal sympathetic nerve activity and renal blood flow during natural behavior in rats. *Am. J. Physiol.*, 286: R881–R887.

Zamboni, G., Perez, E. and Amici, R. (1997). Biochemical approach to the wake–sleep cycle. In: Lugaresi, E. and Parmeggiani, P.L. (eds). *Somatic and Autonomic Regulation of Sleep*. Berlin: Springer, 3–24.

Zamboni, G., Amici, R. Perez, E., *et al.* (2001). Pattern of REM sleep occurrence in continuous darkness following the exposure to low ambient temperature in the rat. *Behav. Brain Res.*, 122: 25–32.

Zepelin, H. (2000). Mammalian sleep. In: Kryger, M.H., Roth, T. and Dement, W.C. (eds). *Principles and Practice of Sleep Medicine*. Philadelphia: Saunders, 82–92.

Zepelin, H., Siegel, J.M. and Tobler, I. (2005). Mammalian sleep. In: Kryger, M.H., Roth, T. and Dement, W.C. (eds). *Principles and Practice of Sleep Medicine*. Philadelphia: Elsevier Saunders, 91–100.

Zinkowska, S.M., Rodriguez, E.K. and Kirby, D.A. (1996). Coronary and total peripheral resistance changes during sleep in a porcine model. *Am. J. Physiol.*, 270: H723–H729.

Zoccoli, G., Bach, V., Cianci, T., *et al.* (1994). Brain blood flow and extracerebral carotid circulation during sleep in rat. *Brain Res.*, 641: 46–50.

Zoccoli, G., Andreoli, E., Bojic, T., *et al.* (2001). Central and baroreflex control of heart rate during the wake–sleep cycle in rat. *Sleep*, 24: 753–758.

Index